FROM BIRTH TO MATURITY

Founded by C. K. Ogden

The International Library of Psychology

DEVELOPMENTAL PSYCHOLOGY
In 32 Volumes

FROM BIRTH TO MATURITY

An Outline of the Psychological Development of the Child

CHARLOTTE BÜHLER

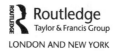

Routledge
Taylor & Francis Group

LONDON AND NEW YORK

First published in 1935 by
Routledge

Reprinted in 1999, 2000, 2001 by
Routledge

2 Park Square, Milton Park, Abingdon, Oxon, OX14 4RN

Simultaneously published in the USA and Canada by Routledge

711 Third Avenue, New York, NY 10017

Transferred to Digital Printing 2007

Routledge is an imprint of the Taylor & Francis Group

First issued in paperback 2013

© 1935 Charlotte Bühler
Translated from the German by Esther and William Menaker

The publishers have made every effort to contact authors/copyright holders
of the works reprinted in the *International Library of Psychology*.
This has not been possible in every case, however, and we would
welcome correspondence from those individuals/companies
we have been unable to trace.

These reprints are taken from original copies of each book. In many cases
the condition of these originals is not perfect. The publisher has gone to
great lengths to ensure the quality of these reprints, but wishes to point
out that certain characteristics of the original copies will, of necessity, be
apparent in reprints thereof.

British Library Cataloguing in Publication Data
A CIP catalogue record for this book
is available from the British Library

From Birth to Maturity
ISBN 978-0-415-20985-4 (hbk)
ISBN 978-0-415-86439-8 (pbk)

CONTENTS

LIST OF PLATES

vii

ACKNOWLEDGEMENTS

A SERIES of lectures under the auspices of the New Education Fellowship and later in the Froebel Institute and in different Universities and Colleges in England was the original basis of this little book. It has grown since then through additional material, mainly from Continental and English literature, and is a kind of integration of a great many details which have been collected. It is hoped at some later date to make use of the abundance of American material now available. The book has been written so that *teachers* and *parents* as well as *students* may make use of it.

I wish to dedicate this little book to my co-workers, to all those who for years have been striving, together with me, toward the same scientific goals ; to those whose friendship, enthusiasm and help have been of inestimable value for me and my work.

I can enumerate only a few, those who helped with this little volume. In making my special acknowledgements, I wish first of all to mention *Dr. Lotte Danzinger* and *Dr. Liselotte Frankl*, to whose unceasing efforts I owe much of my material ; *Dr. Maria Maudry* and *Dr. Emmy Sylvester*, who helped me in gathering the literature ; *Dr. Hertha Herzog*, who compiled the statistical data, and *Drs. William* and *Esther Menaker*, who made every effort to provide a careful translation. I want also to thank *Dr. Käthe Wolf*, who set up the index ; *Ms. Leopoldine Plischke* and *Mr. Rudolph Gröger*, who contributed the drawings, *Miss Agnes Bondy*, head nurse of the Kinderübernahmstelle in Vienna, who contributed photographs ; *Dr. Pearl Greenberg* and *Dr. Ellen Nora Ryan*, who helped me with the proofs and the final set-up of the book. I wish also to thank *Professor Dr. Hildegard Hetzer*, who gave me much of her as yet unpublished new material.

CHARLOTTE BÜHLER.

NEW YORK,
February 1935.

INTRODUCTION

THE development of modern child psychology in the last ten to twenty years, through its systematic study of the child in all its life situations, enables us to-day, not only to present a very complete *scientific picture* of mental development, but also to solve many of the *practical problems* which children present. Psychology can now give us information and advice in regard to those practical problems that confront parents and teachers in the understanding, upbringing and education of children. It can in addition assist us in meeting such community problems as the care, placement and treatment of orphans, children of the poor, feeble-minded, delinquent, adopted and foster children. The study of the *development of the normal, average child* has given us a *standard of comparison* and a basis for understanding the mentally ill, the delinquent, the retarded and the problem child. It is therefore important for the public and for all those who work with children to be informed about the normal mental development of the child, and to make use of the help which child psychology offers.

Ever since *Alfred Binet* for the first time made

tests of feeble-minded children, it has been the aim of child psychology to prove itself as useful and indispensable to practical life, as physics is to technical science. The success of child psychology has in this respect been hitherto very limited. Whether the failure of applied child psychology was due to a premature attempt to translate theory into practice, to an approach that was too crude, or whether the complexity of the subject made its application particularly difficult—at any rate, the results left much to be desired. The various test systems, some of which were based on the work of *Binet*, and others that were independently worked out, were applied on a large scale only in America, and even there met with considerable opposition. In spite of the care and circumspection with which *William Stern, Ovide Decroly*, and *Cyril Burt* have used these tests, the prevailing attitude in Europe is still a sceptical one. The psychotherapists among the physicians, who concerned themselves with the psychic difficulties of children, with the exception of the most recent contributors in that field, as for example *Curt Boenheim* of *Erich Benjamin*, have for the most part rejected the findings of child psychology as unusable. They have drawn exclusively either on the psychoanalytic teachings of *Sigmund Freud* and his followers, or on the Individual Psychology of *Alfred Adler*.

A far-reaching change is now under way. It is becoming ever clearer that the achievements of modern child psychology which have grown out of the experimental investigations of the last two decades, are producing results which are of great practical significance for the educator, social worker and physician. The tests for small children (pre-school children) based on ten years of study, enable us to recognize with certainty *psychic abnormalities or retardations, as early as the end of the first half-year.* We are also in a position to make *evaluations of the personality of the one- and two-year-old child*, which are of decisive significance in establishing its suitability for *adoption.* We can also determine whether or not the environment is having a favourable effect on the child, thus enabling us to advise parents and educators as early as the first year. We can pass judgment on the efficacy of methods of upbringing and estimate their effects on the child ; we can achieve an insight into the causes of various types of school failures and ascertain degrees of maturity and ability ; we can form an accurate picture of the effects of institutional upbringing, of the nature of the relationship between child and foster mother and of the suitability of the foster mother.

An attempt will be made in the chapters that follow, to present in precise and succinct form the most important facts concerning the psychic development of the normal, average child. Special emphasis will be laid upon those of the above-mentioned results which are of outstanding practical importance. Since our researches in Vienna represent a ten-year period of systematic study of the total development of the child and adolescent, our own data will, as a matter of course, furnish the basis for this volume. We will, however, also avail ourselves of the outstanding literature in the field.

FROM BIRTH TO MATURITY

SECTION A

THE PRE-SCHOOL CHILD

CHAPTER I

INVENTORY OF THE FIRST YEAR OF LIFE

As a result of our observations and experiments, we are in possession of an especially clear orientation in regard to the first year of life. We were able to establish for the first year of life a more complete and inclusive inventory than we have been able to set up for any of the later age-levels. We employed the method of continuous observation to achieve this inventory and supplemented it with numerous experiments devoted to special problems. *Wladimir Bechterew* [1] in Russia and *Arnold Gesell* [2] in America were the first to apply the method of continuous inventory to the study of individual children. Shortly afterwards in Vienna we made a study of 60 infants, observing them for 24 hours continuously, and in this way

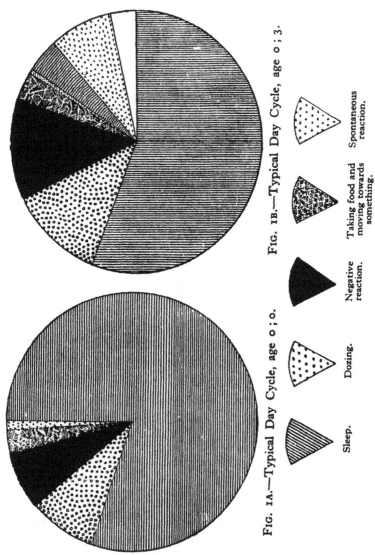

FIG. 1B.—Typical Day Cycle, age 0 ; 3.

FIG. 1A.—Typical Day Cycle, age 0 ; 0.

Sleep.

Dozing.

Negative reaction.

Taking food and moving towards something.

Spontaneous reaction.

FIG. 1.—Distribution of Total

2

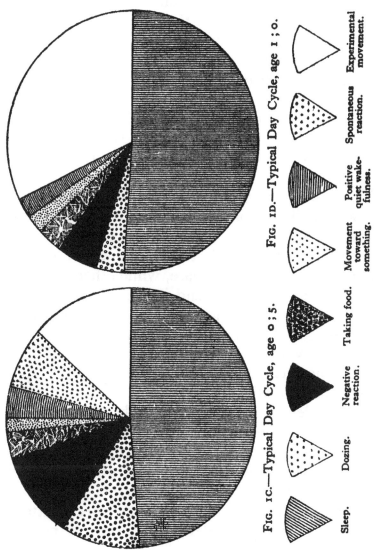

FIG. 1D.—Typical Day Cycle, age 1 ; 0.

Experimental movement.

Spontaneous reaction.

Positive quiet wakefulness.

Movement toward something.

FIG. 1C.—Typical Day Cycle, age 0 ; 5.

Taking food.

Negative reaction.

Dozing.

Sleep.

Daily Behaviour : "Day Cycles." [4]

got a perspective of the entire first year.[3]   At first glance it was clear that modes of behaviour grouped themselves so that each age-level showed a characteristic distribution. The preceeding chart presents this distribution in the course of one day graphically.

Each of the circles represents a 24-hour day ; each sector a time-span within that day.   The size of the sectors indicates the average distribution of types of behaviour within the day. The cross-section was arrived at by studying five healthy children for each month of the first year for one day and night.   Tables I and II show us the regularity with which the frequency of certain behaviour patterns decrease, while others increase during the first year ; and it becomes clear from the average that we get from relatively few individuals, that there is a fundamental law of development at work.   The tables on the next page show the average time intervals for the main types of behaviour within the day.

The development is especially clear in the diminishing sleep needs of the child.   The child of one year resembles the adult more closely in this respect than the new-born infant.   In the course of the first year most parents who are at all concerned with the child pay special attention to its sleep.   Later this interest is not so general.

Several investigators have attempted to set up the minimum sleep period necessary for children

4

TABLE I

Average Times for the Main Types of Behaviour in Minutes

Age	Sleep and Dozing	Negative Reaction	Positive Reaction	Spontaneous Reaction	Sum in Minutes
0 ; 0	1,275	104	47	14	1,440
0 ; 1	1,106	237	73	24	1,440
0 ; 2	1,031	187	89	133	1,440
0 ; 3	979	179	121	161	1,440
0 ; 4	1,051	171	124	94	1,440
0 ; 5	848	159	129	304	1,440
0 ; 6	883	122	126	309	1,440
0 ; 7	826	146	93	375	1,440
0 ; 8	849	99	155	337	1,440
0 ; 9	814	83	113	430	1,440
0 ; 10	712	101	135	492	1,440
0 ; 11	780	57	93	510	1,440
1 ; 0	791	77	112	460	1,440

TABLE II

Reaction Groups in Percentage of the Whole Duration of the Day

Age	Sleep and Dozing	Negative Reactions	Positive Reactions	Spontaneous Activity	Sum in %
0 ; 0	88·7	7·0	3·3	1·0	100
0 ; 3	68·8	12·0	8·2	11·0	100
0 ; 6	56·1	8·4	8·5	27·0	100
0 ; 9	57·0	7·3	7·7	28·0	100
1 ; 0	55·0	6·4	7·6	31·0	100

at different age-levels. The following table gives an average of their findings.[5]

TABLE III

MINIMUM AMOUNT OF SLEEP REQUIRED FOR CHILDREN AND ADOLESCENTS

1- 2 years	.	.	.	13–16	hours
1- 3 ,,	.	.	.	12–15	,,
3- 4 ,,	.	.	.	12–14	,,
4- 5 ,,	.	.	.	11–13	,,
5- 6 ,,	.	.	.	11–12	,,
6- 9 ,,	.	.	.	10–11	,,
10-17 ,,	.	.	.	9–10	,,
15-19 ,,	.	.	.	8- 9	,,

Y. Kamimura,[5a] in a statistical study of several thousand children from 4 to 15 years, found that only 21–23 per cent got the amount of sleep that he had set up as necessary. Most of the children as a result of neglect slept too little. An American questionnaire, carried out with mothers by *Anderson*, *Foster* and *Goodenough*,[5b] revealed a similar condition.

We differentiate further three large behaviour groups, the positive, negative, and spontaneous reactions. Positive and negative reactions are movements toward or away from stimuli ; spontaneous movements are those that occur independent of any ascertainable external stimuli. The reactions directed toward stimuli in the new-born child are first of all those movements that take place during feeding ; later, listening, looking, grasping ; in short, positive responses to stimuli arising in the environment. The new-born child reacts to most external stimuli negatively, i.e. with flight and shock responses, since it cannot as yet assimilate powerful sound and light stimuli. The majority of its reactions are as yet negative. In the course of the first year, however, the negative responses are increasingly replaced by positive ones. We can say that the child learns to assimilate and master the influences arising out of its environment, whereas in the beginning it was overpowered by them. The following chart shows us this development.

External stimuli constantly upset the balance of the child

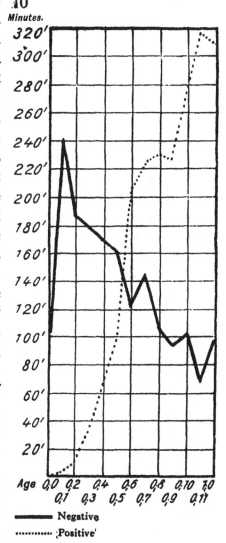

Minutes.

——— Negative

············ Positive

FIG. 2.—Positive and Negative Expressional Movements in the First Year of Life.

7

during the first six months, but in the course of its second half-year the child learns to maintain its balance in the face of the impact of the world around it. When the child begins at the end of its first year to walk and to explore its surroundings independently, its equilibrium is again disturbed, upset, endangered. We find as a result that the second-to-fourth-year-old child is thrown very easily out of equilibrium and that only with the fifth and sixth year of life is it again regained.

The most interesting types of behaviour that occur during the first year of life are the spontaneous reactions. They are, as a matter of fact, not reactions, i.e. they are not at any rate reactions to external stimuli. We know from *Jennings'* researches on protozoa that these spontaneous movements can be observed in all living organisms earlier than specific responses to external stimuli, and that they are reactions to internal stimuli that drive the individual organism to free movements.

Just as the amoeba spontaneously extends its pseudopodia in all directions, the new-born baby impulsively moves its arms and legs in all directions. In the course of the first year these apparently purposeless movements are replaced by investigatory activity with material ; these in turn later give way to creative activity with material. The purposeless movements we call functional organ activity, and we find that functional activity together with exploration are the corner-stone for the future creative activity of the species. Exploratory movements appear as early as the second month. The infant plays with its own fingers, moves and observes them simultaneously. The child makes use of the exploratory movements with play material in the fourth month, and we can already at this age discern individual differences inasmuch as some children show a large and others a small repertoire of manipulations when playing with a rattle or cloth. It is indeed possible that talent and imagination find expression at this early age in the diversity of play movements.

The spontaneous movements become predominant during the first year. They represent 1 per cent of the new-born infant's total activity. Within the first year, however, they increase to 30 per cent of all the activities and more than two-thirds of the responses while awake. This fact alone indicates their importance for the development of the child.

CHAPTER II

TESTING MATURATION IN THE PRE-SCHOOL AGE

IN order to test the maturity of the child in all of its dimensions, we cannot confine ourselves to those large behaviour groups that we have already discussed, but must extend our tests in many additional directions. Our tests are applied to six different fields of activity : namely, the sensory responses, body control, social behaviour, learning and imitation, activities applied to material, and intellectual performance. In two chapters that follow, maturity as manifested in the spheres of social behaviour and activities with material, perhaps the two most important behaviour groups, will be presented in detail. In this chapter the results of our tests in all the six above-mentioned behaviour groups will be given. An exhaustive description and explanation of the tests that we have developed during the ten years of experimental study can be found in the book, *Testing Children's Development.*[6] A short explanation of our system follows.

Our test system differs radically in its point of departure from most psychological tests that are used to-day, including the *Binet-Simon* tests, with the single exception of the *Gesell* tests.

Most test systems are set up in the following manner : the reaction of several thousand children to a given task is tested. The suitability of each task for a given age-level is then statistically established. This procedure neglects entirely the psychological connotations of the tested behaviour in relationship to the development of the child. Let us assume that as a test problem a six-year-old child is asked to define the word " knife ". The question arises, is the ability to define intrinsic for the child's mental development at this age level ? It is from this point of view that we approach the problem of testing. We test only those activities that we have already established as characteristic expressions for a specific level of development. We can consequently determine the extent to which a child is advanced or retarded and can make a psychological diagnosis, on the basis of which we can predict and advise. The following example should serve to illustrate the subtle psychological details that our test procedure utilizes for diagnosis.

We give to each of the four infants, A, B, C, and D, ages 1 year to 1 year 3 months (1 ; 0–1 ; 3), two sticks that can be fitted into each other. We know from our studies of infants of this age that the characteristic response in the manipulation of objects is to bring two things in contact with each other. We expect then that the two sticks will be brought in contact by rubbing or hitting. The manipulation of two objects simultaneously is the characteristic moment in this performance and the bringing of the two objects together furnishes the basis for many complex patterns that are later acquired.

Let us see how our four infants behave. " A " does nothing with the sticks, looks at them without touching them. He is passive. A comparison of this response with those in other test situations will make it possible for us to determine whether the child is unable or unwilling to occupy himself with this particular material and otherwise normal, or whether he is passive in all of his reactions. In the latter case, either a characterological tendency manifests itself in all the test responses or the child is timid, afraid of objects as a result of a lack of experience. This would mean that he is a neglected child not used to having toys.

Infant " B " takes both sticks, rubs and hits one against the other, i.e. his behaviour fulfils our expectations. He is normal.

Infant " C " takes one stick, waves it and strikes other objects with it. This response is that of a child of six months and implies, therefore, a retardation of six months.

Infant " D " takes both sticks and places them so that they form a continuous line. This response is somewhat advanced since it is preliminary to the next stage in which the sticks are fitted into each other.

A detailed description of our interpretative procedure illustrated by individual cases will follow.

It will show that these tests have a practical value for parents, teachers, physicians and social workers. They aid in the diagnosis of behaviour problems, retardation, and exceptional ability in children, and help in making decisions regarding institution or foster home placement and adoption. We are further able to distinguish in cases of retardation whether the cause is environmental or endogenous, and in many cases can give constructive advice.

Some examples from our test series will serve now as illustrations. The following are the tests for the third, fourth, and fifth month:

Psychological Dimension	3rd Month	4th Month	5th Month
Intellectual activity	—	—	—
Manipulation of material	—	Holding rattle	Moving one plaything
Social responses	Babbling Answering the look of adult with smile or babbling	— Reaction to breaking off of contact	— Following a moving person with the eye
Learning	Persisting look after disappearance of object	Noticing change in adult's face created by mask	Reaction to the novelty of situation when carried about
Body control	Producing and observing of own movements	Moving arms and legs when lying face down	Lifting head and shoulders with assistance when lying on back
	Holding up head when lying face down	Holding up head and shoulders when lying face down	Lying face down supported only on palms of hands

Psychological Dimension	3rd Month	4th Month	5th Month
Body control	Listening to noise of rattle when lying face down	Following moving object with eye when lying face down	Removal of obstacle through adequate body control
	—	—	Stretching out arms toward object
	—	—	Grasping object already touched
Sensory perception	—	Examining parts of object successively	—
	Following moving object with eye	Touching object	Holding and looking at object simultaneously
	Looking around when carried	Reaction to simultaneous optic stimuli	—
	Staring at distant object	Searching for source of sound with eyes	Looking at coloured cardboard longer than at uncoloured one
	Turning head inquiringly for source of sound	—	—

A child is tested not only with the test series for his age, but also with the series for the two preceding months and the two months that follow. The test results are evaluated quantitatively as well as qualitatively. The quantitative result is expressed as D.Q., that is, developmental quotient. This quotient represents the relationship between the developmental age (D.A.) and the chronological age (C.A.). A qualitative interpretation can be arrived at through an analysis of the performances in the different psychological dimensions. A concrete example will illustrate the method.

QUANTITATIVE EVALUATION

G. 3000, 0 ; 4 + 0 *

Test	4th Month 0 ; 3–0 ; 3+29	5th Month 0 ; 4–0 ; 4+29	6th Month 0 ; 5–0 ; 5+29	7th Month 0 ; 6–0 ; 6+29
10	+	+	–	–
9	+	+	–	–
8	+	–	–	–
7	+	+	–	–
6	+	+	–	–
5	+	+	+	–
4	–	+	+	–
3	+	+	+	+
2	+	+	–	–
1	+	–	–	–
Problem solved	9	8	3	1
Problem unsolved	1	2	7	9

$$D.A. = 0 ; 4 - 1 \times 3 \text{ days} + 8 \times 3 \text{ days} + 3 \times 3 \text{ days} + 1 \times 3 \text{ days}$$
$$= 0 ; 4 - 3 \text{ ,, } + 24 \text{ ,, } + 9 \text{ ,, } + 3 \text{ ,,}$$
$$= 0 ; 4 + 33 \text{ days}$$
$$= 0 ; 5 + 3 \text{ days}$$

$$D.Q. = \frac{D.A.}{C.A.} = \frac{0 ; 5 + 3}{0 ; 4 + 0} = \frac{153}{120} = 1 \cdot 27$$

* This means that the child is 0 years 4 months and 0 days old.

Thus far the test gives us a purely quantitative evaluation. We see that this child is somewhat ahead of her age group and know that this advancement is characteristic for the average middle-class child.[6a] This is, however, not sufficient. We want to determine as accurately as possible in just what directions she is advanced and what the causes for this advancement are. That is, we want to arrive at a qualitative as well as a quantitative interpretation of her developmental level. In order to present graphically the qualitative differences in the various fields of performance, we have worked out a diagram which gives us what we have called the developmental profile.

We see at a glance that while the child is normal in respect to sensory and social responses, she is advanced in memory reactions, manipulation of materials and body control, i.e. physical and mental development are better than average. We can enlarge our qualitative estimate from our general observation of the child. A trained observer, by comparing the child's performance in the test situation with those of other children, can supplement the qualitative data furnished by the tests. While this additional data gives us some insight into characterological variations, it is gained as a result of accurate observation rather than as a result of measurement. In order to establish tests for qualitative behaviour differences we are now working out devices for their registration.[7] This is of great psychological importance because we can frequently in this way uncover the factors that are responsible for advancement

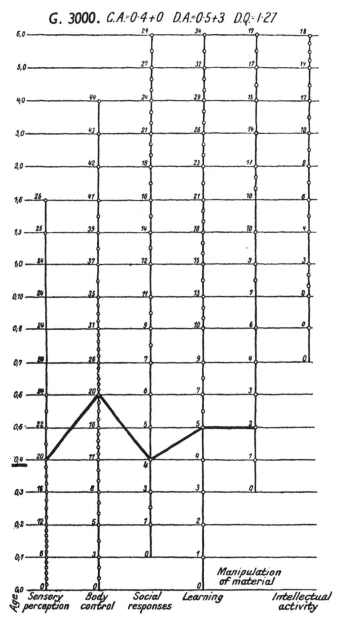

FIG. 3.—The Developmental Profile.

or retardation. Some of the important fundamental personality differences that are brought out in the child's response to the total test situation are activity or passivity, concentration and persistence or flightiness and lack of application. Keeping these qualitative criteria in mind we would characterize the child as follows :

The child's development in every psychological dimension is not equal. She is most advanced physically. Good performance also in material activity and learning. Sensory reception and social behaviour correspond to her age-level. The child is able to grasp objects and can free herself from a diaper put over her head. This response is characteristic for 5-month-old children. Successful body control and the efficient grasping of objects are due not only to the good physical development of the child, but also to her general activity. During the test she never lies quietly in her bed, but is constantly moving about. She shows a great interest in things, as well as in the situation as a whole, and while lying in bed raises her head in order to see better.

The child lacks persistence both in the manipulation of material and in the social situation. If a toy is taken away from her, she makes no objection but soon finds something else to play with. When alone she plays with one toy only for a short period of time. Her lack of persistence is also evidenced by the fact that she fails to follow people moving about the room with her eyes. This comparatively bad development of sensory activity can be explained by the child's general unrest.

The child was already advanced when two months old. This is clear from the distribution

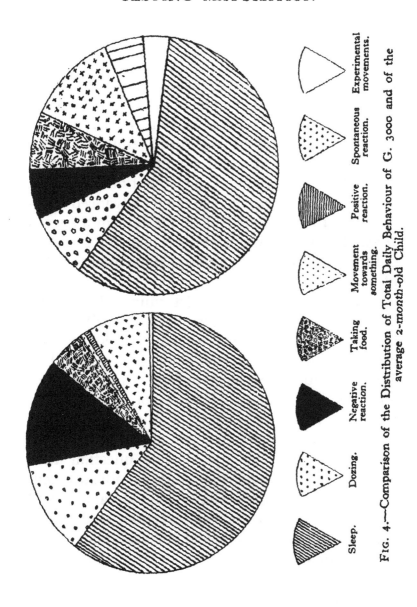

Fig. 4.—Comparison of the Distribution of Total Daily Behaviour of G. 3000 and of the average 2-month-old Child.

Experimental movements.

Spontaneous reaction.

Positive reaction.

Movement towards something.

Taking food.

Negative reaction.

Dozing.

Sleep.

of her total daily behaviour which we arrived at through a 24-hour observation of her at that time. This distribution is represented graphically by the circle on the page before.

G. 3000 is an example of a well-developed, advanced child. This advancement is typical of pre-school children of well-to-do families. They are physically well cared for and receive stimulation through toys and the attention of adults. *Maria Wolf*[8] has investigated advanced pre-school children of well-to-do families in a special research study to which we shall turn our attention before discussing the opposite phenomenon, that of retardation.

It was first necessary to determine whether the same test materials could be used with these children which we had already employed with poorer children. We found that it was possible. We had anticipated large differences in performance but found that they were not so great as to preclude the possibility of a quantitative comparison. We established for these children an average quotient of 130.* The question then arose as to the particular kind of advancement which these children show. As we anticipated (see Fig. 5), they showed exceptional development in the manipulation of material and speech performances, the two fields in which they actu-

---

* This same average quotient is, since the work of *Lewis Terman*,[8a] generally accepted also in intelligence tests with well-to-do children. See also more recently *M. Shirley*.[8b].

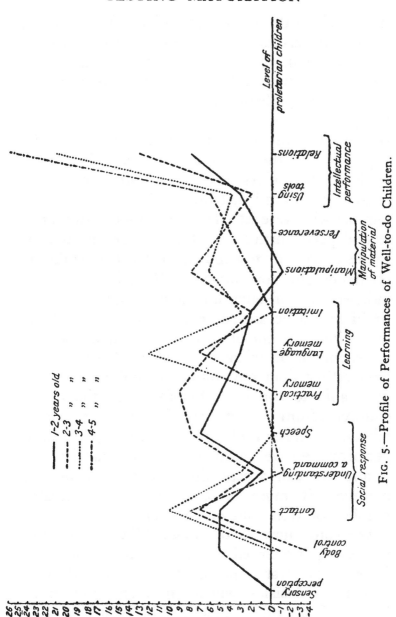

FIG. 5.—Profile of Performances of Well-to-do Children.

ally received the most stimulation. In two other fields our results were the opposite of what we had expected. First of all these children who were especially well developed physically achieved only average performance in body control, whereas the performance of the neglected children in this respect was relatively superior. This may be explained by the fact that they are called upon to help themselves to a much greater extent. Second, we found that the children of well-to-do families who were tested showed much better intellectual performance than the average, in spite of the fact that our test indicated that this ability is relatively (in comparison with other abilities) independent of environmental influences. The problems to be solved required practical intelligence independent of speech ; i.e. their solution is dependent on talent or intellectual precociousness rather than environmental influences. We were able to conclude therefore that the tested children from better-class homes were more talented than the proletarian children upon whose performances we based our test standardization. Before we can accept this result as definitive, however, it must be checked with a greater number of tests and of children.

We come now to the most difficult problem, the testing of retarded children. The psychologist faces his greatest responsibility when called upon to make a decision which can colour the entire future of a child. Practical problems of this nature will be discussed in the following chapter. At this point we will present our findings in a few additional cases together with our interpretations.

The boy B. 1834, with the chronological age of 1 ; 4 + 24, the developmental age of 1 ; 2 + 3 and the developmental quotient of 0.83, is more than two months retarded. From an analysis of his developmental profile (Fig. 6) we arrive at the qualitative structure of his mental level. It becomes clear from the chart that his social development is very good, that his sensory reactivity is normal, but that he is retarded in all other respects, especially in his intellectual activity.

Our test should enable us to decide what the causes of this retardation are, and how it can be corrected. There are two major possibilities that should be considered. The original endowment of the child may be inferior, or the environment itself may lack the variety of stimuli that the child needs to achieve normal development. There is in addition a third possibility, namely that the retardation may have a neurotic basis. When there is lack of original equipment we cannot speak of retardation but rather of native insufficiency. When the environmental factors alone are responsible for the difficulty we may use the term retardation. In the case of neurosis, the performance is neither insufficient nor retarded, but inadequate. The neurotic child's unnatural reactions are determined in part by harmful environmental influences, in part by constitutional

CASE 1 : RETARDATION AS A RESULT OF CONGENITAL DEFICIENCY
B. 1834, 1 : 4 + 24 *

Psychological Dimensions	9-10 Mon.	11-12 Mon.	2nd Year 1st Quarter	2nd Year 2nd Quarter
Intellectual activity	Everything +	(10) Getting object from behind screen. — (9) Investigating parts of bell. + (8) Getting hold of object by means of string. —	(10) Reaching for biscuit in mirror. —	(10) Remembering under which of two boxes a biscuit has been placed. — (9) Showing preference for figured cardboard to plain one. +
Manipulation of material		(7) Opening box. + (6) Carefully holding hollow blocks together. +	(9) Filling and emptying out hollow blocks. —	
Learning		(5) Imitating adult's ringing of bell. — (4) Remembering contents of box after 1 min. +	(8) Imitating adult's squeezing of ball with chicken.† — (7) Remembering chicken in ball after 3 min. + (6) Remembering contents of box	(8) Drumming with two sticks after seeing adult do it. — (7) Remembering disappearance of chicken into ball after 8 min. — (6) Remembering contents of box

Social responses

(3) Turning to adult in astonishment. +

(5) Understanding a command. +

(3) Turning to adult in astonishment. +

(5) Understanding that something is forbidden. +

(4) Organized game with ball. +

(4) Turning to grown-up for information. +

Body control

(2) Standing up with support. +

(3) Holding something while walking with support. +

(3) Holding something while standing without support. −

(1) Getting up into sitting position. +

(2) Standing without support. −

(2) Walking without support. −

Sensory perception

(1) Rubbing and hitting sticks together and listening. −

(1) Watching spinning top. +

$$\text{D.A.} = 1;3 - 18 - 45 + 36 = 1;2 + 3$$
$$1;3 - 6 \times 3 - 9 \times 5 + 9 \times 4 = 1;2 + 3$$
$$(0;11,\ 0;12)\ (1;0 - 1;3)\ (1;3 - 1;6)$$
$$\text{D.Q.} = 0;83$$

* Means Boy, number 1834 among our cases, aged 1 year 4 months and 24 days. G. would mean Girl.

† A rubber ball out of which a rubber chicken appears when it is squeezed.

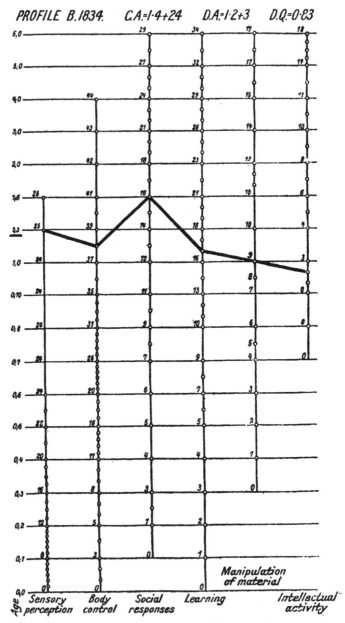

FIG. 6.—Developmental Profile of B. 1834.

factors. Not much can be done in the case of congenital deficiency. Lack of stimulation can be corrected by environmental control and direction. The neurotic child requires careful psychotherapy. It is of the greatest importance, therefore, that in every case which presents a deviation from the normal, the cause of the deviation be correctly determined. A quantitative interpretation of the test results is insufficient as an indicator for causes and treatment. The mere change of certain environmental influences would be completely inadequate in the case of a neurosis. whereas a psychotherapeutic treatment of the child would be unnecessary in the case of native insufficiency or retardation. We shall try to make these differences as clear as possible by discussing several cases in detail.

In the case of the child under discussion, we find that he is retarded in the manipulation of material. It is possible that the child lacks experience of this kind, that is, that he has not been given enough toys. It is also possible that the child lacks initiative and has on this account little experience with material objects. The latter interpretation (namely, that the child lacks initiative) is confirmed by the fact that the child is also retarded intellectually and that his responses during the tests were unusually passive and slow. This lack of initiative is further substantiated by the fact that the child did well in all those tests which required no spontaneous activity but are initiated by a command from the adult. (Game with partner or carrying out a command.) On the other hand, the child fails in all the tests that necessitate a certain amount of activity (getting an object from behind a mirror, finding a biscuit under boxes, filling and emptying hollow blocks, etc.). The possibility still remains that this shyness, passivity, and lack of initiative is not an innate, inborn deficiency but an outgrowth of environmental influences, i.e. neurotic reactions. The child's normal social responses do not, however, support this assumption. Mistakes in upbringing influence social behaviour first and foremost, and neurotic patterns resulting from the poor upbringing manifest themselves most clearly in social responses. Where the child's social behaviour is normal we can conclude with almost absolute certainty that we are not dealing with a neurosis. As we progress in our analysis of this child's test it becomes ever clearer that he has a congenital mental defect. It would, however, be more accurate perhaps to speak of a lack of ability here, rather than of definitive feeble-mindedness. This lack of ability is reinforced by a constitutional passivity. The fact that in cases of feeble-mindedness we encounter poor intellectual performance, coupled with good social behaviour, lends weight to this interpretation. Feeble-minded children are sometimes so highly social that they are considered extremely intelligent by ignorant parents who confuse lively social behaviour with intelligence.

Whereas the test results of the above case led us to the conclusion that the retardation of two months was largely congenital, the following case will illustrate a much greater retardation that is entirely the result of environmental influences.

CASE 3. G. 1713, 1 ; 6 + o, is a girl who until two months preceding our test had been in an institution. During the period of institutionalization the child was physically well cared for but its psychic needs were entirely neglected. The child spent its last two months there quarantined because an infectious disease was suspected.

It is obvious that this child is unusually backward. A quantitative calculation of the developmental age gives us 1 ; 0 + 18, i.e. a retardation of more than 6 months. The unevenness, however, of the child's performances in various fields would seem to indicate that the developmental quotient is not reliable. On examining the child's performances carefully we find that the child fails in all the tests for one year or over. The child was then retrogressively tested as far back as the sixth month and even failed in several of the sixth-month tests. The distribution of the + and − shows us that the most consistent deficiency exists in social responses. Five of the seven social tests for 6–12-month children were negative for this 1½-year-old child. What does this signify? One might assume that the child is congenitally feeble-minded and more or less incapable of social reactions. This is not substantiated, however, by the child's performance in the fields of intellectual activity, memory, and the manipulation of material, all of which achieve the 12-month level. Furthermore, as we have said before, the social response is generally highly developed among feeble-minded children. One might assume in the second place that there is a neurotic involvement. Injurious environmental influences reinforced by repeated failure and a possible constitutional predisposition, lead to neurotic reaction patterns that manifest themselves unmistakably in the social situation. The retardation in so many other fields, however, does not lend strength to this assumption. Neurotic children as a rule are not only highly intelligent but are seldom as intellectually retarded as this child who shows a retardation of a half a year.

Just as we often find good social reactions coupled with poor intellectual activity in feeble-minded children, so we find on the other hand good intelligence coupled with poor social performance in neurotic children. A third type of retardation is that conditioned by the environment. Such a milieu does not, as in the case of the neurosis, create difficulties for the child because it establishes conflict, but the neglect to which the child is subjected is responsible for retardation in all directions. The child is shy because it is not accustomed to friendly contact

TESTING MATURATION

G. 1713, 1 ; 6 + o

Psychological Dimensions	6th Month	7th Month
Intellectual activity	—	—
Manipulation of material	(10) Holding on to toy when attempt is made to take it away. +	(10) Hitting a toy against a stationary object. +
Learning	(9) Anticipating event which has often been experienced in the past. + (8) Negative reaction when toy is taken away. +	(9) Imitating grown-up's beating on table. + (8) Searching for lost toy. +
Social responses	(7) Mimicking friendly or angry expression. —	(7) Initiating social contact. +
Body control	(6) Sitting up with help. + (5) Raising head and shoulders when lying on back. + (4) Freeing self from diaper over head, when lying on back. — (3) Grasping something with one hand. +	(6) Turning on side from back position. + (5) Sitting up with support. + (4) Freeing self from diaper when lying face down. — (3) Turning for object when sitting with support. +
Sensory perception	(2) Distinguishing between doll and bottle. — (1) Selective fixation of object from its surroundings. +	(2) Reaching for light. + (1) Grasping for edge of table. +

31

G. 1713, 1; 6 + 0

Psychological Dimensions	8 Months	9 and 10 Months	11 and 12 Months	1 ; 0–1 ; 3
Intellectual activity			(10) Getting object from behind a screen. – (9) Investigating parts of bell. + (8) Getting hold of object by means of string. +	Everything –
Manipulation of material	(10) Getting toy by changing body position. + (9) Moving two toys about. +	(10) Choosing between two toys. +	(7) Opening box. + (6) Holding hollow blocks together carefully. +	
Learning	(8) Retrieving toy from grown-up's pocket. –	(9) Hitting two spoons together. + (8) Drumming with one stick after seeing adult do it. + (7) Uncovering a hidden toy. +	(5) Imitating grown-up's ringing of bell. + (4) Remembering contents of box after 1 min. +	

| Social responses | (7) Organized game of hide and seek. + | (6) Attracting grown-up's attention. − | (3) Turning to grown-up in astonishment. − |
| | (6) Taking toy away from grown-up. − | (5) Responding adequately to gestures. − | |

Body control	(5) Moving about. +	(4) Creeping. −	(2) Standing up with support. −
	(4) Staying in sitting position by holding on. +	(3) Sitting without support. +	(1) Getting up into sitting position. −
	(3) Pushing grown-up's hand away when nose is being cleaned. −	(2) Freeing self from diaper while sitting without support. −	
	(2) Freeing self from diaper on head when sitting with support. −	(1) Grasping for two toys while sitting without support. +	
	(1) Reaching for object outside of bed. +		

with grown-ups. It cannot handle material because it has had no experience of that kind, and has been given no toys. Because of neglect it is physically underdeveloped and its body control is therefore poor. This general retardation, in turn, influences the child's intellectual development unfavourably. In contrast to the feeble-minded child, however, it does not show a deficiency in intellectual activity which exceeds the deficiencies in all other fields.

Let us now consider the environment of the child under discussion. It comes from an institution where there were almost no play opportunities and only very minimal contact with grown-ups. These factors alone would suffice to explain the child's low-grade social response. Why, however, is the child's response to material inadequate?

In the test situation this child's initial response both to toys and to the examiner was one of shock. The child cried and sat motionless in front of the toys. In the course of the next $2\frac{1}{2}$ hours, being left alone, it gradually became accustomed to the toys and carried out some of the movements that we expect from a child of its age. We find this sort of response among those children who have no opportunities to play with toys, who find neither encouragement nor stimulation in their surroundings and who require several hours in the test situation before they can overcome their psychic inertia, and respond to the stimuli that are presented. This capacity to achieve performances in the course of the test situation, of which they were at first entirely incapable, is characteristic of neglected children.

The same phenomenon may be observed in the children of more primitive peoples. Our tests were applied to Albanian children [9] with practically the same results. The Albanian children grow up not only without playthings, but in general play much less than our children. In so far as they play at all, their games are mainly social, a reflection in all probability of the importance of social activity among primitives. Their play with material things on the other hand is very limited and one-sided. The Albanian children are kept in a completely darkened room to protect them against malarial infection, and are bound fast in their cradles so that they are deprived of all opportunity for either bodily or sensory activity (Photo 1, plate I, Albanian baby in the cradle and unbound). Just as in the case of our neglected children, these children accustom themselves to play material in the course of a few hours and within that time go through the same series of stages, for the completion of which our normal children require several months. In the course of time they produce manipulative movements characteristic of the various age-levels, although they lack the skill, ingenuity and variety present in the productions of a normal child.

It becomes clear, therefore, that our tests are designed to isolate those reactions that are prim arily the result of inherent maturation from those successful performances that are a result of practice or training, since those children who have had no experience whatsoever with material cover the preceding phases of activity in a short habituation period and achieve the same degree of maturity in response as the children who have had unlimited experience. These tests were also the first that could be successfully applied to negro children.[10] Their aim is to test the level of maturity that the human organism has achieved, independent of environmental and cultural influences, at any rate as far as the pre-school child is concerned.

The above case was that of a child who suffered psychic injury and retardation as a result of complete neglect and indifference on the part of its environment. The neurotic child presents a third type of retardation. We will discuss as third case that of G. 1869, chronological age, $4 ; 4 + 0$.

G. 1869. C.A. $4 ; 4 + 0$

Psychological Dimensions	4th Year	5th Year
Intellectual activity—	(10) Understanding a picture. +	(10) Putting a jumping jack together. +
(Comprehension of the relationship between form and meaning) (Use of tools)	(9) Removing an object that is attached to a hook by a ring. +	(9) Using a matador hammer as a tool. +

PLATE I

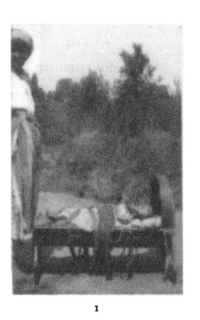

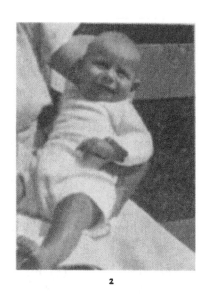

1

2

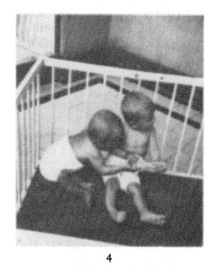

3

4

1. Albanian Baby in the Cradle and Unbound.   2. Smiling Reaction.
3. Offering of a Toy to another Child.   4. Taking Away and Defending of a Toy.

[face p. 36

Psychological Dimensions	4th Year	5th Year
Manipulation of Material— (Perseverance)		(8) Game requiring patience. + (Getting *one* mouse into a trap)
(Making something out of material)	(8) Naming something built out of blocks. —	(7) Naming a drawing. —
Learning— (Imitation)	(7) Copying circle. +	(6) Copying diagrammatic drawings. —
(Verbal memory)	(6) Reciting verse of 8 syllables and 3 numbers. +	(5) Reciting verse of 12 syllables and 4 numbers.—
(Practical memory)	(5) Finding 3 out of 4 hidden things. +	(4) Finding 4 out of 5 hidden things. —
Social Responses— (Speech)	(4) Telling about some plans. +	
(Invitation)	(3) Sorting 200 slips of paper after one request. +	(3) Carrying out 3 orders. —
(Contact)	(2) Evaluating an act that is described according to usual moral principles. +	(2) Competing in a game. — (1) Observing rules of a game. —
Body control	(1) Carrying a container filled with water. +	

The test sheet shows that all of the child's intellectual performances are normal for its age. An absolute interpretation of the general level of the child's total performances and the developmental age could not be established, as the child refused to carry out many of the tests. Out of the seven social tests only five were carried out ; of these five, three were negative. We have here great social retardation combined with well-integrated intellectual activity. The child also fails in just those tests that require the manipulation of materials simultaneously with the establishing of contact with another person, for instance when the child is asked to name something it has built or drawn, or asked to copy someone else's drawing or to repeat a verse, etc. The child handled materials in the test situation only when the adults present withdrew from the immediate vicinity. The child's actual developmental age could not be determined, since we are justified in assuming that its performances would be much better once its inhibitions had been overcome.

It is characteristic for the neurotic child that social inhibitions indirectly limit its performances in other fields.

The child's general behaviour and history substantiate our test finding. At the time of the test, the child was placed for the second time in an institution. The child's behaviour was quite normal at the time that it was separated from its family for the first time and placed in a foster home. Two months later when removed from the foster home it had changed completely. According to the records of the institution, the foster home was unsatisfactory and the child was removed on the recommendation of the social worker. Unfortunately the record furnished us with no information as to why the foster home was unsuitable. We must conclude, however, from the change in the child's behaviour that the experiences of these two months had been highly traumatic and had left a deep impression on the child. On returning to the institution for the second time the child avoided every possible contact with adults and allowed itself to be touched only under violent protest. When the child thought itself unobserved, however, it tyrannized over the other children. At the beginning of the test the child ran into a corner of a balcony and refused to play with the offered materials, and only after the other children began to interest themselves in the play materials did it edge up to the group and show some interest in the toys. After the child had been left alone for some time it began to build with some blocks.

The three cases under discussion should serve to illustrate our method of interpretation in the practical application of our tests. Before proceeding to the scientific formulation regarding development in childhood and adolescence, we will include a chapter that will demonstrate the practical advice and guidance that we are in a position to give on the basis of our test results.

CHAPTER III

PRACTICAL APPLICATIONS

OUR tests are of practical value for two large groups of cases. To the first group belong those children whom we generally designate as problem children, that is, children who are unable to adjust themselves to their environment. As a result their parents, teachers, or guardians are forced to seek the aid of the psychologist in order to get advice regarding methods of upbringing that will correct the difficulty. To this group also belong those children who present no special problems, but whose parents seek information about their general development in order to discover the child's weaknesses before it is too late, and to correct them if possible. To the second group belong those children who for one reason or another must be placed outside their own homes. This includes children who are privately adopted, but more especially, the vast majority of public charges, i.e. children who are removed from a delinquent and pauperized family situation or orphans who must be provided for by the community. In such cases a psychological diagnosis should enable us to determine whether the child is to be recommended for adoption, for foster home or institutional placement or for medical care. In those countries where the harmfulness of institutional upbringing has already been recognized, it is the general opinion that for normal children, at any rate, placement in foster families is the best solution of the problem. It is important, however, that the suitability of the foster family be psychologically established. The cases that follow illustrate our practical procedure. The first two are private cases that involve complicated problems in upbringing.

NEUROSIS. B. 14, 4 ; 0. Child is brought to the physician because he refuses to urinate in the standing position. The physician diagnoses the difficulty as a neurosis and wants to know if our test furnishes any special indications. The test gave the following picture. The level of the child's performance is somewhat below that which we expect from a child of this age who comes from a comfortably situated family. An examination of the test details reveals very uneven performances in the various fields of activity. The child's speech development and memory are normal, but he can solve only those problems that require theoretical intelligence. The test for the manipulation of materials is entirely negative. In this respect the child is almost two years retarded, since he handles material like a 1–2-year-old child. Those problems also for the solution of which the skill of the two-year-old suffices, remain unsolved.

One might assume that this is a child who is theoretically talented but lacking in practical ability. It is possible that a congenital lack of skill is responsible for the child's retarded performance in the material manipulation tests. Our test finding, however, in other fields of performance do not substantiate this simple interpretation. In its social responses, although the child is not absolutely negative, it fails in exactly those tests that investigate the child's maturity in regard to the relationship to other individuals and to the group. The child avoids any problem that demands the slightest patience or exertion. This would seem to indicate that lack of skill in the handling of materials does not suffice to explain this child's unusual retardation in this respect. The difficulty is much more the result of a lack of will and patience. This lack in combination with anti-social attitudes would seem to indicate that there is no congenital defect, but rather deficiency, i.e. the child is in conflict with its environment. A conflict of this kind is an indication of neurosis. It is nevertheless quite possible that the predisposing cause for this neurotic involvement is a primary lack of skill in the handling of material that has been reinforced by an over-solicitous and protective environment. This was clearly brought out during the test situation since the child appealed constantly to someone in the environment for assistance. An interview with the mother confirmed this behaviour trend that we observed in the test situation. In this case we advised psychotherapy.

NEUROSIS. The next case presents a similar but simpler problem. B. 1871, 4 ; 5 is a boy who was brought to us because of the following difficulty : The relationship between the parents is bad ; they quarrel constantly about the child. The father wants us to approve of his methods of upbringing and to confirm the fact that the child is unusually well developed for its age.

Our test revealed that the child's speech and intelligence were very highly developed, but that in all the other fields of activity its performance was no better than average because it failed in those tests that required patience and persistence. The one-sided intellectual development of this child as well as his lack of patience and persistence are danger signals for his future development and may already be indications of a neurosis. Our observations made during the test situation confirm this assumption. The child is neither willing nor able to content himself with the same material for any length of time and demands a constant change of playthings. If they are not forthcoming at once, he plagues everyone in his environment. This child lacks not only the patience and concentration necessary for the solution of a problem, but also control in his response to the experimenter who is a total stranger to him. We learn that in spite of the child's mental alertness and dexterity, he is unable either to dress himself or to eat alone, and is in constant need of help. It is possible that we are dealing here with an inherent lack of patience in regard to the solution of both purely intellectual and practical problems, that has been strengthened by his parents, since the child's conduct is almost always defended by one parent when criticized by the other. The recommendation in this case was that the child be sent to a kindergarten, so as to avoid, in part at any rate, the witnessing of parental differences, and in order to accustom it to independent and persistent occupation.

We have not as yet succeeded in diagnosing all the forms of neurosis with our tests since these tests are primarily designed to set up developmental rather than characterological data. We are at present working on a series of tests that are calculated to give us characterological information independent of developmental factors. The utmost care, however, must be exercised in the interpretation of test results. They enable us, when interpreted conservatively, to arrive at a crosssection of the child's psychic developmental level. It is possible to reach specific conclusions regarding the origin and cause of the modes of behaviour tested, because we are acquainted with the conditions that generally favour their development. Notwithstanding, a given test result may be determined in a variety of ways and it is necessary therefore not to rely exclusively on the test results. We need in addition a reliable personal history and a detailed description of the child's environment. The following case should serve to illustrate the impossibility of evaluating the child's psychic developmental level without such additional information :

No Definite Diagnosis Possible. G. 1859, 1 ; 8 was placed in an institution for a time, as the mother had to go to a hospital and there was no one at home to care for the child. The nurses were struck by the fact that the child remained shy and unapproachable for a much longer period than usual. They considered the child definitely backward and brought it to be tested.

Our results showed that the child was normal in every respect with the exception of social responses, where it failed completely. Since we have, as mentioned above, found that children who test well intellectually and poorly socially are neurotic, the conclusion would lie near at hand that the same is true in this case. The solution of this problem, however, was complicated by the following elements :

1. The child had never before lived in a situation away from its pleasant and comfortable home. It is possible that the transfer to an institutional environment was therefore more of a shock than it usually is for children whose homes are not exceptionally good.

2. This child stands on the threshold of a phase (second year) that is usually characterized by negative attitudes towards strangers and novel experiences.

We are therefore not in a position in this case to make a definite statement until we have found out from the mother if and when difficulties of this nature have first made their appearance. This information will also have to be carefully evaluated inasmuch as we know that in the course of the second year all children go through a social crisis, so that in this case if the difficulty is of recent origin we may be dealing with a transient normal condition. If we learn, however, that the child was abnormally shy and quiet as early as the first year, the chances are that the child's social behaviour is an expression of an innate character tendency. Should no more data be available to explain this social inhibition, it would seem advisable to withhold a final diagnosis for another six months, since the crisis that the child is experiencing makes an exact interpretation very difficult.

SPECIAL DEFECT. The next case is much simpler psychologically than the two that preceded, and presents the problem of retarded development in one specific direction. G. 1896, a little girl of chronological age 2 ; 10, was brought to us because she had not yet learned to speak and the parents were anxious to know whether the defect was developmentally or organically conditioned. The final diagnosis in this case should be made by a physician ; we can only, with the aid of our tests, prepare the way by establishing the child's developmental level. The test revealed that intellect, memory, manipulation of materials and dexterity were exceptionally well developed, i.e. the child's performance was better than average in all those tests that did not require an understanding and mastery of speech. Since in addition there were no signs of neurotic involvement present, the child was sent to a speech correction clinic, where the case was diagnosed as acoustic aphasia.

The following are not child guidance cases, but involve the question of child placement.

OBSTINACY, NO DEFINITE DIAGNOSIS. G. 1687, chronological age, 3 ; 4. This child was returned to the city authorities by its foster parents because they could not cope with the difficult behaviour problems which it presented. It was necessary to determine through the test whether the child was abnormally stubborn, i.e. neurotic and therefore not suited to foster home care, or whether it should be transferred to another foster family.

It was found that the child was very well developed as far as intellectual activity, bodily control and manipulation of materials were concerned. Its language and social development, on the other hand, were no better than average, although the child was in no sense retarded. It is quite possible that the foster family in which the child was placed did not meet the child's intellectual and social needs, and that a lack of understanding stimulated conflict. Good intelligence accompanied by average language and social responses might point to a neurotic tendency. We find some confirmation for this diagnosis from our observations of the child's test responses. Once the child became interested in some test material, it refused absolutely to be diverted by the activity of, or the materials offered by grown-ups. Since the child was on the other hand very active, ingenious and persistent, the concentration of interest on very few objects might be interpreted as a sign of unusual talent, and perseverance. It would be necessary to study the child carefully over a period of several hours in order to determine whether the child's absorption in play was the result of stubbornness or special abilities.

We advised that the child be placed in an institution long enough for it to outgrow the stubbornness resulting from unintelligent upbringing and also to give it more time to itself. It could then later be placed in a carefully selected, intelligent foster family. It is occasionally necessary, with difficulties of this kind, to advise removal of the child from its own home if the parents are either unable to learn or if the methods of upbringing are definitely harmful.

FEEBLE-MINDEDNESS. In conclusion, the two cases of feeble-mindedness that follow should serve to show how a psychological consultation regarding the same problem can lead to different corrective measures. Both B. 1894, C.A. 2 ; 1 + 2 and B. 1575, C.A. 1 ; 10, are such clear cases of retardation that it would be obvious to any layman. We were called upon to decide whether they should be placed in a foster family or in an institution. Experience has demonstrated that certain of the milder forms of feeble-mindedness thrive best when placed with simple families where the adaptation does not require high-grade intelligence, while the more serious forms of feeble-mindedness can only be cared for in an institution.

B. 1894 is not only retarded, but he is also sick. He is a congenital syphilitic and has already had three courses of treatment. As a result he is so retarded physically that his bodily control is only that of a twelve-month-old child. In addition, he is so retarded intellectually that he can solve none of the twelve-month problems ; he fails in all the social tests that require an understanding of language and those that require a certain amount of activity. He shows, however, considerable manual dexterity in playing with materials, and more capacity for imitation than in any other direction. His memory performances are those of a child of 1 ; 6. A powerful imitative drive combined with an almost complete absence of intellectual comprehension occurs frequently in serious cases of feeble-mindedness.

It became clear from the child's responses in the test situation that he belonged to the excitable type of feeble-mindedness. He cried aloud and reacted with powerful effect in various situations, and was not to be diverted or quieted.

We recommended further medical examination

and institutional placement since the degree and kind of feeble-mindedness rule out the possibility of family placement.

FEEBLE-MINDEDNESS. Let us now turn our attention to B. 1575. All of this child's intellectual performances were negative ; all his social responses positive. Imitation with and manipulation of materials was lacking, but memory was good. Since the child was in an institution until a short time before the test its deficiencies with material may be the result of institutional neglect. It is possible that if properly cared for this child's intellectual responses will improve.

We advised placement in a carefully selected foster family in which the child's intellectual inferiority would not create any difficulties.

SUMMARY

Our test experience led us to three major conclusions :

First, we achieve a picture of the child's total psychological level and development by testing the child in a series of typical performances, which are indicators for the psychological structure of its personality.

Second, an analysis of the positive and negative test results supplemented by general observation of the child during the test situation as well as by its social history enables us to throw some light on the possible causes of deviations from the normal. We differentiate the following factors :

A. Endogenous variants. These occur as precociousness, retardation, presence or absence of special abilities. Inherent deficiencies such as feeble-mindedness also belong in this category. A diagnosis of this difficulty can frequently be made as early as the first year.

B. Variants resulting from environmental influences. These variations from the norm can be precipitated either by a lack of interest and encouragement on the part of the environment and therefore furnish a basis for retardation, or by especially favourable and positively stimulating environmental factors and therefore result in precocious development. It is possible to recognize those variations from the norm that are caused by neglect, that is, a complete absence of opportunity to use those functions that are developing, and those that are produced by careful upbringing and ample and satisfying stimuli.

C. Variants resulting indirectly from environmental influences. These variations from the norm are the result of the interaction of characterological predispositions in the individual and specific environmental influences causing a neurosis.

Third, the following indications for corrective measures may be arrived at from the total personality picture and the test diagnosis :

(a) In cases of children who are retarded, defective, or precocious in a given direction, a change in the kind of stimulation offered as well as opportunity for the exercise of specific functions can serve either to raise the general level of performance, or to create compensations for deficiencies. In cases of feeble-mindedness, for example, that are diagnosed early, memory training can overcome to some extent inherent deficiencies. A child whose speech development is advanced for its age, but whose ability to manipulate material is poor, can, through special practice in this field, be kept from a one-sided development. In the case of defectives, the child must either be referred to a physician or placed in a suitable institution.

(*b*) Change or supervision of environment can serve as a corrective measure in many cases. The study of environmental factors and their effect on the child has led us to recommend the removal of children from their own unsuitable homes to good foster families, to advise families in methods of upbringing and to suggest reform measures for institutions.

(*c*) In cases of neurosis, psychotherapeutic treatment is indicated.

CHAPTER IV

SOCIAL DEVELOPMENT IN THE PRE-SCHOOL AGE

THE development of the child's relationship to other human beings involves some of the most difficult and fundamental problems of child psychology. Research in this field has begun only within the last decade.

The greatest difficulty lay in finding a suitable method for the study of the problem. Two possible models were at hand in the fields of psychiatry and animal psychology.

Modern psychiatric study of the neuroses rather than the psychoses has revealed that relationships with other human beings experienced by the child can be of decisive etiological importance in the neuroses. The psychic content of these relationships both conscious and unconscious were therefore carefully studied. *Sigmund Freud*, who did pioneer work in this direction, set up a psychological system that explains the development and structure of human relationships. He differentiates a positive and negative component and designates the positive component as sexuality, the negative one as aggression or destruction. These components, their origin, their developmental stages, their combination with one another, their outward manifestations were all arrived at through an analytic study of human experiences.

53

THE PRE-SCHOOL CHILD

A method for the study of social responses that is diametrically opposed is that used in animal psychology. Here objective behaviour rather than subjective experience is investigated. *David Katz* was the first to approach the problem systematically. He set up objective criteria for studying the social behaviour of chickens. Observations made on chicken farms of thousands of chickens enabled him to make definite statements regarding their social behaviour. Offensive, defensive and submissive behaviour were distinguished and the domination of some individuals as well as the inferior position of others was established.

Similar studies were made in Vienna with school children at the suggestion of *Karl Bühler*. It was found that this method of approach could also be successfully used in the field of child psychology.

In 1924 we applied this objective method for the study of behaviour patterns to an investigation of the beginnings of social responses in infants. We tried to establish clearly the appearance of the first contact, i.e. to set up definite criteria for the first specific reaction to other human beings. The responses of children to one another was also studied. In America and Germany research on the social responses of children was carried out in this manner, so that we now possess an extensive literature. On the basis of all of these results we will present a picture of the development of social reactions in children. Later, we will go into problems of interpretation and into some of those questions which psychoanalysis has raised.

The question arises, how can the earliest reaction of the new-born child to other human beings exactly be determined ? During the first four to five weeks of its life the infant's reactions to external stimuli consist of reactions to loud noises, strong optical stimuli or direct and violent handling of its body. There is no response to stimuli of low intensity. The child reacts to powerful stimuli with shock. Toward the end of the first month and the beginning of the second, specialization takes place in the reaction to different sounds, and different optical stimuli. At the same time the first specific reaction to another human being appears. The child smiles when spoken to (Photo 2, plate I, Smiling reaction). Three studies have proven definitely that the child's first smile is a primary and specific social reaction. Only later does smiling occur in response to other situations and stimuli, such as tickling or the presentation of toys.

It is of the greatest psychological significance that the infant's first reaction to other human beings is a definitely positive one. The child's negative social responses are a secondary development. Throughout the first year of life positive social behaviour predominates unless the environment is very unfavourable.

Differentiation of these positive social responses begins at a very early age. At five months the child becomes socially active, i.e. it seeks contact spontaneously with those who approach him, both by making sounds (babbling) and by physical contact (grasping and touching). At six and seven months the infant tries eagerly to include anyone who is present in its play. Objects are given and received from others and the child enjoys especially those games that include a partner, hide and seek, exchange of toys, etc. (Photo 3, plate I, Offering object ; Photo 5, plate II, Community of play). The partner's gestures are observed at the latest in the fifth month and at eight months there is an astonishing capacity for interpreting and understanding them. Children of this age have been observed trying to comfort a frightened or crying child. On the other hand, we have also recorded situations in which one child did everything possible to exclude and subdue its partner, and at ten months such behaviour has been accompanied by triumphant smiling.

This brings us to the manifestations of negative social behaviour. They include flight, defence and attack, and are secondary reactions. During the first year there are two factors that condition flight and defence responses : interference and strangeness. Aggressive behaviour is usually produced by the sight of a desired object in the possession of another person.

The new-born infant reacts to an interference with its freedom of movement with cries and violent movement of the entire body. If a child's hands or feet are held fast, or an attempt is made to deprive it of a toy, every effort is made to regain bodily freedom or the toy. On the other hand, a six-month-old child will attempt to take a plaything away from another child if he is eagerly interested in a toy (Photo 4, Plate I,

Plate II

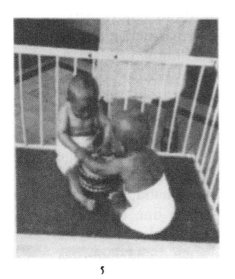

5

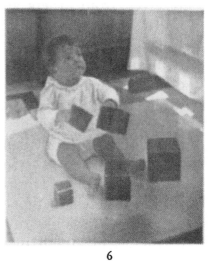

6

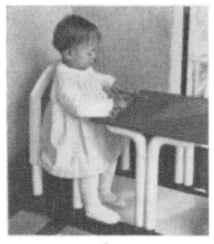

7

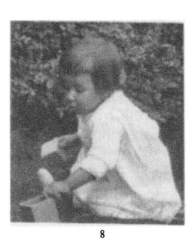

8

5. Community Play.   6. Boy 1 ; 0 shakes two Hollow Blocks and hits one against the other.

7. Boy 1 ; 3 rubs two Sticks one against the other.   8. Girl 1 ; 4 carefully places down Hollow Bricks.

Taking away and defence of object). Defence against interference or an aggressive act set in motion by the desire for an object are reactions which to a certain extent are only incidentally directed towards people. The child pays no attention to the playmate and is dominated exclusively either by the desire to get free or to get or retain a specific toy. It is then by the last third of the first year that the child expresses satisfaction and pleasure in triumphing over a rival, that is to say, he is then becoming aware of the effect which his dominance of the situation creates. In research that is under way, we are attempting to get an accurate picture of the superiority reactions and the specific triumphant smile that we find in children about ten months old.

Individual differences in play situations of this kind are very marked. There are children who are so aggressive that they are interested in any object another child may have in its hand and attempt to get possession of it at once. Then there are those children who are definitely on the defensive, who never of their own accord interfere with another child but who either defend themselves against attack or take flight.

The following protocol, made during the first study of this type of behaviour, is given as an illustration. A very aggressive eight-month-old child is playing with a child of ten months, who defends itself against the attacks of the younger one.[11]

Herber C. 0 ; 10 + 17 with Elaine Q. 0 ; 8 + 3

H. has the doll which is lying in the play pen.	E. reaches for it, first with right then with left hand.
H. retreats.	She is annoyed and energetically reaches for the doll.
H. holds the doll up in the air and looks at the experimenter.	She makes a third attempt to get the doll.
H. resists holding fast with all his might.	She looks at the doll.
H. plays with the doll ; handles it.	She tries again to take the doll away from him . . .

Unfamiliarity of another person is the second factor responsible for flight and defence reactions. During the first year the child's response to strange impressions is preponderantly negative. Once the child begins to perceive individual details its reaction to change is immediately negative. For instance, if a five-month-old child is accustomed only to seeing a person full face and suddenly sees him for the first time in profile, it reacts with fear. It gets frightened, cries, and looks for the second eye. An unfamiliar grimace, such as knitting of the brow, a new hat, or a radical change of dress, can frighten a six-month-old child and stimulate a negative reaction even to familiar individuals. At the age of about a year, strangers are distinguished from familiar individuals and also call forth negative responses. This attitude towards strangers gets stronger and persists until about three years of age, when the social responses become very involved and emotional.

Personal emotional reactions are the fourth conditioning factor responsible for negative or positive social behaviour. Thus far research that has been done in this field would seem to indicate that subjective sympathy or antipathy for definite persons does not appear before the second year. In the first year, for instance, we cannot observe a preference for certain individuals with the exception of mother or nurse, that is, the most familiar person. From the second year on the favouring of definite individuals becomes the most characteristic feature of the child's reaction to people and it remains so until about 4 or 5 years.

By observing the behaviour of the child we can find out the content of this preferential response. From the end of the second year on we see a type of response to others that is best described as ardent. This includes not only ardent preference but also violent dislike for certain individuals. The child manifests its affection by caresses and fond words, and indirectly by offering assistance and giving presents. Frequent seeking for contact, clinging to a favourite when there is a prospect of separation, flight to him in danger, and jealous reaction when someone else approaches, are signs of a strong positive response. In cases of violent negative response we observe hitting, pushing away, antagonistic expressions such as " you're bad ", rejection of friendly overtures, help or bodily contact with a given individual, flight and asking the person to go away. Responses of this nature can be either constant to a specific individual or fluctuating to various individuals. It has been observed, for example, that on a certain day a child takes flight from an unpleasant situation and runs to its mother, and regards all the other members of the family with antagonism, but that on the following day it selects someone else as a protector and includes the mother in the group that it dislikes. Hatred of a person who is generally the object of affection can also appear on occasion.

> Dietrich, 4 ; 5. His father, of whom he is ordinarily very fond, punishes him for disobedience. Sobbing, he runs out of the room : " Mother, we have no father any more. That man belongs to Grandpa." The child, lacking another weapon, thinks and wishes the father out of the family.

This singling out of those who are especially liked or disliked can be conditioned from without and varies. Still it cannot be denied that certain individuals are the preferred objects of great love and devotion. On the basis of child behaviour observed from the second year of life on, it is possible to speak of love and hate reactions for which we can set up definite criteria. *Freud's* psychoanalytical school has attempted to discover the genesis and content of these love and hate reactions by application of its analytic method. That is, an attempt is made to bring forgotten childhood memories into consciousness so that the patient can re-experience them in their original form. We believe that a discussion of psycho-analytic results will become valuable only after we can make comparisons between the data found by the psychoanalytic method and the data found by the method of direct observation of children's behaviour.

As yet we are only in a position to come to a conclusion in regard to social behaviour during the first year. We have established objectively that the friendly and antagonistic behaviour patterns that occur during the first year differ radically from those of the second. With the exception of those members of the immediate family (including nurses) with whom the child comes in very frequent contact, the child does not as yet differentiate between individuals. The child smiles, babbles and makes physical contact with everyone. Flight and defence are caused by unfamiliar behaviour and interference with freedom of movement. As we have mentioned previously, neither sympathy nor antipathy, nor ardent responses are as yet manifested. It is of objective significance, however, that social re-actions differ so widely from the first to the second year, that we can assume a fundamental psycho-biologic change. The primary effect of other people on the child is positive and sets in motion an attempt to make a contact. Since it appears as early as the end of the first month it is naturally a very primitive response and quite different from the powerful devotion that is observed in the second year. We are not as yet in a position to say what the intrinsic character of the first effect of others on the child is.

The objective psychologist must be wary of interpretations at this point. We see that the child's primary reaction pattern is a positive movement towards, and a smiling at the adult.

In contradistinction to objective psychology, psychoanalysis introduces at this point a specific theory and interpretation. According to the theory a drive called libido propels the child towards other people. This positive response is interpreted as the effect of libido and as a tender affectionate movement towards other people. This drive towards others the analysts connect with pleasurable bodily stimuli which the child receives from others through contact, etc., i.e. the child moves positively toward those from whom it receives pleasurable stimuli.

How is one to conceive of a transferred response of this kind ? At the early age under discussion—a child smiles at another human being at the age of one month —we can only speak of a transference of this nature as similar in structure to the conditioned reflex. A transfer of responses of this kind can be observed in the feeding situation where the $1\frac{1}{2}$-month-old infant reacts with the same suckling movements which it makes when something is brought in contact with its mouth, when it is placed in the accustomed position on its mother's arm. The significance of this early transference of reactions lies in the fact that an original reaction pattern is repeated in response to a new stimulus. In the case of the smiling of the child, however, we have to do with a reaction for which there was no prototype. On the contrary, smiling, which is primarily a social response, is later transferred to other situations. We must conclude, there-fore, that the primary response of the child to people is a totally different one from its response to things and situations and we cannot speak of transferred reactions in the former case as we can in the latter.

The contention of psychoanalysis that all positive reactions to other human beings are of a sexual nature, dilutes and generalizes the term sexual to such an extent that it becomes unspecific in its meaning. A term of this sort is of restricted value for the empirical scientist, since its application is so broad that it makes finer differentiation impossible. The objective psychologist observes that the infant in the first year smiles at all other human beings, that at the end of the first year and during the second year the child reacts positively only to familiar persons, that after the fourth month familiar persons become increasingly differentiated from strange ones, that from the second to the fourth year an extreme dependence upon specific individuals arises, and that this response can be clearly distinguished from the simple positive responses, etc. An ever-increasing specialization and intensification of the positive reactions takes place, which finally become concentrated on one individual after having gone through phases in which all human beings, then familiar individuals and finally the most familiar person are recipients of the positive responses. In this last phase the parents and other individuals begin to have a specific significance for the child. A systematic study of the psychic patterns involved in this process is one of the most important problems with which we are at present concerned.*

* The Psychological Institute of Vienna with the aid of the Rockefeller Foundation has begun an extended study of the child in the family situation. Further information regarding this project can be found on pages 208 *ff.*

Thus the facts as objectively observed are as follows :
In the first place, in the second to the fourth year of
life, the child's reaction to other people becomes quite
different from what it was in the first year of life.   The
problem now arises as to the nature of these reactions.
But before any interpretation can be offered, a second
important observational fact has to be stated.   This
observation relates to masturbation in early infancy
and to the circumstances under which masturbation
takes place in the first year of life, that is to say, so
far as it takes place at all in this early period.   Even
so far as this is a fact, the opinions differ.   The
opinion of the psychoanalyst, *J. K. Friedjung*,[11a] is
that this is a normal and everyday occurrence.   *C.
Boenheim*,[11b] the pediatrician who collected a large
body of observations in the Berlin Polyclinic, considers masturbation, in early childhood, a sign of
prematurity and degeneracy.   No matter which opinion
may be correct, we must state the following essential
fact.   That is, all observational material shows that
the masturbative manipulations of infants occurs
regardless of who is or is not present, and has no
connection with the presence of the preferred person.
Small children masturbate when they are left to
themselves in a play situation, sometimes with someone present.   This seems to indicate that these
physical enjoyments of the body's pleasurable functions
have nothing to do with emotional reactions to people,
but are a development in quite another direction.
In fact, one of the great difficulties of adolescent
masturbation is the effort to unite these two trends,
the physical and the emotional, which are normally
separate.[11c]

The child begins now, not only to discriminate
between individuals but also to expect consider-

ation as an individual. At this age the child becomes sensitive to the presence or absence of friendliness and attention.

Amy Daniels, directed by *Bird Baldwin*, in an experimental child study of this developmental phase was able to show the far-reaching importance of sympathetic individual care. Two groups of two-year-old children living in the same institution were segregated from each other and subjected to two divergent types of treatment. One group was given very little tenderness although adequately cared for in every other respect. In the other group, a nurse was assigned to each child and there was no lack of tenderness and affection. At the end of half a year the first group was mentally and physically retarded, in comparison with the second. In order to effect normal psychic and physical maturity, individual care and devotion are indispensable in the upbringing of small children.

It is clear that the child needs individual care, particularly at this stage of its development. The removal therefore of children from their homes to institutions is more harmful at this age than at any other. The developing individuality of the child expresses itself not only by its need for individual care, but also in expressions of will and ego-consciousness (self-assertion). This precipitates the first conflicts between the child and its environment.

Our knowledge of the process and dynamics of

personality and will is as yet quite rudimentary. The few facts that we possess will be presented.

A study made by *Ruth Klein* [12] has given us the following insight. If an adult speaks to a one-year-old child in an inviting or forbidding tone, accompanied by the appropriate gestures, the child fails either to understand entirely, or it obeys so immediately that *Klein* speaks of a suggestive effect. Regardless of how we explain or describe this reaction, the fact remains that the responses to a command during the first year, when they take place at all, are as immediate and direct as a stimulus-response pattern. This state of affairs is altered in the second year. The child obeys orders more and more readily since it begins to comprehend them better, but at the same time it shows increasing negative protest responses to a command, even when it obeys. *Ruth Klein* employed simple commands like, " give me that toy," or " stand up," accompanied by an appropriate gesture, and found that towards the end of the second year the child protests against more than half of the orders given, even though they are as yet obeyed. The development of the response to prohibitions follows the same course but appears somewhat later.

The following experiment is very illustrative. The adult forbids the child to touch a toy that is within the child's reach. He then turns away or leaves the room for a moment. All the 1–2-year-olds understand the prohibition as cancelled at the moment that contact with the adult is broken, and play with the toy. If the adult returns suddenly, 60 per cent of the children of 1 ; 4 and 100 per cent of those of 1 ; 6 show the greatest embarrassment, blush, and turn to the adult with a frightened expression. From 1 ; 9 on they attempt to make good what has happened by returning the toy quickly to its place. From two years on they attempt to motivate the disobedience, for example, by claiming the toy as their own. After the age of two the child expresses will, insistence on its own rights, and possessive impulses in its relations with adults.

The first signs of obstinacy, a phenomenon that no childhood lacks entirely, appear in this phase. The differentiation between obstinacy that is at first a normal developmental expression and later becomes neurotic, is one of the important practical questions that child psychology will have to solve in order to enable parents and others who are concerned with the upbringing of children to prevent a transition from normal to neurotic negativism.

We anticipate that the child who is passing through a normal obstinacy phase will express his will, and insist on his rights, thereby encountering the resistance of adults to which it is as yet unable to adapt itself. Or, on the other hand, the adult may make a suggestion to the child that interferes with its own plans, with the result that the child is unable to understand and adjust itself to this complex situation.

> Example : Rolf, 1 ; 8, has just finished his evening meal with his parents, and discovers a new game after leaving the table. He takes two silver serviette rings and puts them on the floor, and then goes into the nursery. The governess keeps him there in order to put him to bed. He cries, and attempts to free himself by force. He is released for a moment, whereupon he runs to get a little broom and carries it to the dining-room. He sweeps the two serviette rings to the other end of the room, then lifts them up from the floor, places them on the table, goes to the nursery with his broom and allows himself to be undressed.

What has taken place here is self-evident. The child had made a plan and was phantasying its execution. An adult interfered in so far as she demanded something entirely different from the child. The child was in all probability not able at this age to accommodate itself to this new situation at once. We see that Rolf was willing to take orders from an adult after his own plan had been realized. It is of course necessary for a child to know that its plans cannot always materialize. In our discussion of the next few months we will no longer consider such difficulties the result of inability but rather of unwillingness, since we expect after a time that the child must learn to accept such situations.

A careful analysis of cases of normal obstinacy reveals, first, that the child is not unwilling but unable to comprehend and master a situation ;

second, that attacks of sheer desperation occur only occasionally, and third, that they disappear after a relatively short period, i.e. a few weeks or months. On the other hand, neurotic obstinacy is characterized by a determined unwillingness to give in ; the attacks occur very frequently and finally the condition can persist potentially for several years. *Erich Benjamin* [13] has investigated carefully a large number of obstinacy attacks of neurotic origin. We cannot substantiate his conclusion that all types of obstinacy answer his description and must be called neurotic. In a study of ours that is being prepared for publication, a large number of cases of obstinacy appear, that resemble those described above and must be called normal.

Florence Goodenough,[13a] who observed, in a very thorough study, the obstinacy attacks of forty-five children in a controlled family situation, also established the normality of this phenomenon since there was not one child who did not at some time or other get into this kind of conflict situation. The ages of the children ranged from 1 ; 6 to 1 ; 10 (there were in addition two children aged 1 ; 11) and in every case obstinacy attacks were observed. The frequency varied from once a week to four times a day. For the normal child this was dependent exclusively on age, as the following curve of Goodenough shows.

It is clear from the figure that obstinacy reaches its highest point during the second year. Although girls at this age level show a greater frequency than the boys, the boys show a stronger predisposition in that direction. After the second year both curves decline rapidly. The curve for the girls shows considerable irregularity between 5 and 7, which is in all probability conditioned by the limited material used.

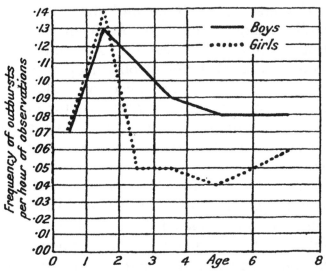

FIG. 7.—The Relation of Age and Sex Differences to Frequency of Obstinacy Attacks. (*After Goodenough.*)

We can conclude that obstinacy attacks are also physically determined from the fact that children who have been ill a great deal are more subject to such outbreaks, and from the fact that children are much more irritable and liable to be obstinate when hungry. The first of these observations was made by *Stratton*, the second by *Gates*, who found that it held good for adults as well.

SOCIAL DEVELOPMENT

It is understandable that only especially severe cases find their way to the clinics. *Benjamin's* claim that since neurotic children are above all obstinate, obstinacy is therefore always a symptom of neurosis, must certainly be considered not as established. Careful analysis of cases shows that the word obstinacy covers a great variety of conditions. Let us compare the above case with the following case of *Benjamin's*.

"Case number 22. H. B., 4 ; 2 years old, has a sister of six. His development during infancy was uneventful ; at eighteen months he had an attack of diarrhoea and presented difficulties from that time on. Intestinal complaints persisted and he gained very little weight. Speech development was delayed and he still is considered behind children of his own age in this respect. H. has been difficult to bring up for some time. Exactly how long his mother cannot say. He does not obey, does just the opposite of what he is asked, is highly excitable and has attacks that are described as " affect respiratory spasms ". It is not definitely known whether laryngeal spasms were also present. He tyrannizes over his mother, is jealous when she does not devote all of her time to him exclusively, and insists on being put on the pot only by her, otherwise he deliberately holds back the passage of stool. He is also jealous of the older sister. He is so easily frightened that one could almost describe it as " nervous " fear. He is afraid of all four-footed animals, of Santa Claus. These anxieties appear in his dreams. He is very restless at home. From his second year on a trembling, especially of the arms, has been noted whenever he is very happy or enraged. Excessive salivation is also present.

THE PRE-SCHOOL CHILD

The youngster is cowardly and afraid to undertake anything on his own. He did not participate in group activities in Kindergarten and played stereotyped games by himself. He soiled himself until the age of three ; masturbated and vomited occasionally.

He is delicate, underweight, has a funnel-shaped breast, and is knock-kneed. When he is at rest a slight tremor is present in the entire body ; it is most marked in the arms and head and is accentuated during periods of excitement. His gait is stiff and ungainly. No signs of organic illness are present ; the findings of a neurological examination were negative.

In the period immediately following his transfer to the institution, the obstinacy attitudes were clearly expressed. He reacted to every request with refusal and a crying attack of long duration. During such phases, his whole body trembled. His general attitude is distrustful. He can do nothing unaided. He can neither feed, nor dress himself, relies entirely on the help of grown-ups, by whom he wants to be spoiled and singled out. He is jealous of the other children ; prefers to play with the two-year-olds, whom he hits on the sly. He avoids children of his own age, inter- feres with their play, but cries when another child approaches him and runs to the grown-ups. If they fail to take his part at once, he gets very much upset. While being washed he clings fearfully to the nurse ; in the gymnasium he begins to cry as soon as he sees the apparatus and doesn't trust himself to approach it. Bed-wetting is intermittent. In general he im- presses one as a much younger child. He stutters, his vocabulary is scanty and sentence structure is primitive. His pronunciation is so distorted and un- clear that he is very difficult to understand. He lisps also.

In the course of four months, the child underwent

a fundamental change. It began with the enjoyment of doing things himself, that in a short time expressed itself as ambitiousness and a wish to help the younger children. His anxieties receded into the background ; he made contacts with the other children, and was soon a great favourite with them. He came out of his shell entirely ; took part in everything and is happy and content most of the time. Although stubbornness does not appear very often his moods change without warning. He still is jealous of children of his own age, wants to be the centre of interest, clings to the grown-ups, plays the " baby ", and attempts to avoid discipline. Excessive salivation and the tremor have disappeared, the speech difficulties have improved considerably. The stammering has been overcome, but the difficulties with sentence structure and lisping are still present. The mother suffers from depressions whose origin has not as yet been determined."

It is obvious in this case that we are not dealing with a normal child. The constant, unmotivated resistance to all requests differentiates this case from normal stubbornness. Then, too, a neurotic mechanism of this kind never appears as an isolated symptom, but always in conjunction with other symptoms such as anxiety, lack of independence, inability to get along with other children, etc. Environmental pressures are usually largely responsible for all types of symptomatic behaviour, including neurotic stubbornness.

A certain degree of self-evaluation is inherent in the independent planning of the two- and three-year-old who begins to hold fast to its goals,

The following scene illustrates this with especial clarity.

> Anna, 3 ; 2, and Eva, who is younger, are alone in the nursery. The parents are near by. Suddenly Eva is heard crying loudly. The anxious parents hurrying into the room learned to their astonishment that Anna had bitten her sister in the finger. Why ? Was it accompanied by effect or was it an accident ? Persistent questioning is of no avail and it looks as if the factors leading to its precipitation will remain a secret. Anna sits on her stool, pale and guilt-laden. She confesses.
>
> For the first time in the child's life the father metes out corporal punishment. Not only that, but the child feels how hurt and mortified the parents are. It is a terrible moment for her. She humbles herself and kisses her father's hand : " Dear father, forgive me, I will never be naughty again." And hopes that, as usual, the father will heed her pleading and forgive. Instead, he demands that she expiate the wrong that she has done the little sister. " Beg Eva's pardon, and everything will then be forgiven." With this the child fell into a boundless fury. Anna sprang up, shouted, raged, threw herself on the floor, got up and cried, her face purple red. " I will ask mamma's pardon ; I'll ask Mitzi to excuse me ; I'll ask Olga (the cook) to excuse me." Anna is willing to ask all the grown-ups' pardon, but she feels that to ask her smaller sister's pardon is an unheard-of insult.[13b]

Unfortunately, we know as yet very little about the entire genesis of the sense of ego in the child. When we consider the crystallization of will that the above cases would seem to indicate, this age must be especially painful for the child, since it is so acutely dependent on the adults in its environment. This actual crisis in the life of the three-year-old must be precipitated by the conflict caused by its dependence on just those individuals against whom the child must at times defend itself and show resistance. *Martha Sturm* in a series of extended observations of small children in the family situation, determined the frequency with which contact between adult and child was

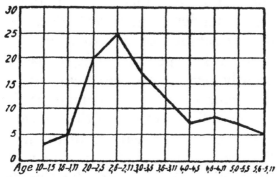

Fig. 8.—Expression of the Desire for Contact.

initiated by one or the other. She found that from the fourth year on the child initiates contacts more frequently than the adult. In the fourth year the child makes more contacts than in any of the other years. The above curve is based on a count made of all those responses that express a child's desire for contact with the adult. Maximal frequency occurs between two and four years.

On analysing the talk of a three-year-old child covering an entire day, we found that about 30 per cent was directed toward the establishment of social contact. This would seem to contradict *Piaget's* statement that the conversation of the pre-school child is exclusively egocentric monologue. Our observations would seem to indicate that *Jean Piaget's* [14] conclusions are correct but incomplete. Undoubtedly the child is egocentric to the extent that his psychic life revolves around his own needs, activities and point of view. He interprets the acts of others in terms of his own motivation. This is a matter of common knowledge. This tendency, however, does not preclude the possibility of a strong drive in the direction of other people. *Piaget* has himself more recently revised his statements in so far as he does not emphasize the monologuous character of the child's talk, so much as the egocentric.

Between five and six years maturing manipulative skill is reflected in a variety of new forms of social behaviour. We can consider this development in detail after we have set up the different stages in the development of the child's manipulation of materials.

CHAPTER V

THE DEVELOPMENT OF THE SMALL CHILD'S RESPONSE TO MATERIALS

THE new-born child closes its hand around an object that touches its palm. This grasp response is entirely reflex and can be understood as a clinging to, rather than a concern with the nature of the object. This clinging, as *J. B. Watson* showed, is strong enough to enable ninety-six new-born children out of a hundred to support their own weight when suspended by the hands.

The earliest finger and hand movements are a primitive form of play without materials. At first the child makes very rapid, later slow movements which it observes and repeats time after time. The new-born infant grasps only in response to contact with an object and gradually, in the course of the fourth and fifth month, the child learns to reach for and grasp an object that it has perceived.

H. M. Halverson [15] has made a careful study of the development of the finger and arm movements employed in grasping. He found that during the first year the finger movements are very rapid and numerous, while the arm movements are very slow. He says that the entire child grasps in this phase. *Edgar Daniels* and *Maria Maudry* [16] in a study of defensive movements in the infant have shown that the characteristic movements are for the second month, hand, then forearm until five months, in the sixth and seventh month the entire arm already.

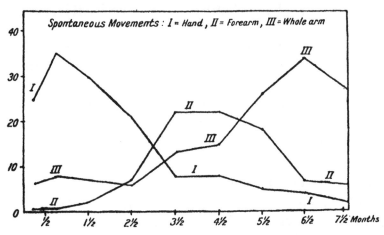

FIG. 9.—Spontaneous Movements. (*After Daniels and Maudry.*)

By the fourth month the child is able to move an object back and forth or rub it against a stationary object. This represents its first experience with materials, the beginning of an activity that is of far-reaching importance in its development and preparation for life. With the exception of the learning of social responses the majority of the child's learning experiences occur in connection with the manipulation of material. We were able to determine the following chronological sequence

78

for manipulative activities. From 4 to 7 months the child handles only one toy ; from 7 months on, two toys. At first objects are shaken (Photo 6, plate II, Two hollow blocks are shaken), then one is rubbed against the other (Photo 7, plate II, Two sticks are rubbed against each other), then hit against one another, then objects are thrown away. Next two surfaces are rubbed against each other. At 10 months the careful putting down of objects follows (Photo 8, plate II, Hollow blocks are carefully placed down) ; at about one year forms are fitted into each other, as, for example, the fitting of hollow blocks into each other (Photos 9, 10, 11, plate III, Hollow blocks and sticks are put one into the other). At the age of $1\frac{1}{2}$ years new forms are constructed by placing one block on another (Photos 12, 13, 14, plate IV, Blocks are put one on the other). Without going into the details of these activities, we can deduce a general law of development. The infant's activities during the first year are characterized by the fact that they are not specific in regard to material, i.e. the child performs the same movements which are characteristic for its level of development regardless of the kind of material with which he is occupied. In one period the child shakes everything ; three weeks later he hits things against one another or throws things away. This is a period in which the child exercises the functions that are developing, on whatever material he is handling. The important thing here is neither the particular material which is used nor the result of the activity, but rather function training (the practice of functions) as such.

At 10 or 11 months the first manifestations of a new type of activity can be noted. The child begins to place objects down carefully, which means that he is no longer merely concerned with his own movements, but that he pays attention to the nature of the material and becomes aware of the effects of his activity upon it. A seven-month-old infant, if given a piece of plasticine, will pat it and wave it around. He will not notice the imprint which his fingers make. Not until the child is 2 to 4 years old does it observe such effects on materials.

A few examples should make clear how the child begins to note the results of his manipulations on plasticine and sand.

M. 168, 2 ; o. Holds a piece of plasticine in her hand and rotates it ; holds on to it firmly ; lays it down ; grasps it again ; rolls it back and forth between both hands ; lays it down ; taps with its fingers ; lifts it up ; drops it ; touches it again ; places both hands on it firmly for a short time ; touches again ; looks at it for some time ; then draws right index finger slowly across the surface (this is a 6-minute protocol).

K. 204, 3 ; o, taps plasticine with right hand ; lifts it up ; puts it down ; touches surface ; rolls it ; presses it out flat ; rolls plasticine into a cylinder ; makes deep holes with fingers.

Predominantly specific manipulation of plasti-

PLATE III

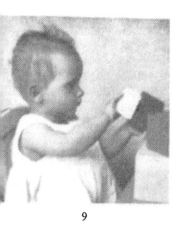

9

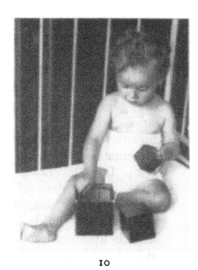

10

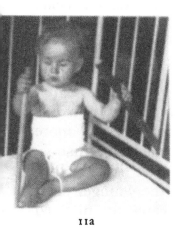

11a

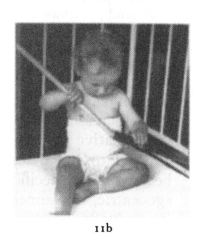

11b

9. Girl 1 ; 4 puts one Hollow Block into the others.   10. Girl 1 ; 10 puts
Hollow Blocks one into the other.

11a. Girl 1 ; 10 puts sticks one into the other.   11b. Same Child, second phase
of Movement.

cine appears for the first time during the fourth
year.

> K. 40, 1 ; 3, is sitting in the sand-pile. Squeezes
> sand between fingers ; hits sand with palm of hand ;
> draws fingers back and forth across sand ; finds a
> stone ; draws it over sand ; takes a piece of wood ;
> throws it away ; crawls around on sand-pile ; reaches
> for small sand-piles ; they crumble when he tries to
> grasp them ; crawls around ; again tries to grasp
> sand ; takes piece of paper ; spreads it out ; crawls
> around ; takes some sand in each hand ; stands up ;
> takes shovel ; holds it upside down ; turns it around ;
> shovels up some sand with it ; throws sand away with
> aid of shovel ; walks around ; throws shovel into
> sand ; pulls it around in the sand ; takes handful
> of sand ; throws it away ; repeats ; walks around ;
> takes some sand ; scatters it around (this is an 11-
> minute protocol).[17]

From the second to the sixth year we see how
the child's treatment of various materials is not
only increasingly specialized but also how his
manipulative techniques become more and more
adapted to the nature of the materials, that is,
become more specific and adequate. The wilful,
egocentric, unplanned attack of the younger child
is gradually replaced by the carefully planned
application of skill.

At about $1\frac{1}{2}$ years a third acquisition in the
child's play behaviour can be observed. The
child perhaps accidentally in playing with two
blocks places one on the other. A younger child
would pay no attention to this. The child of $1\frac{1}{2}$

years suddenly becomes aware of it, its activity is checked and the child contemplates the unintentional product of his play. After a while he may try to pile many blocks, one on top of the other. This done, he will look around with great satisfaction, as if proud of his accomplishment. It is perhaps the first time in his life that he relates his own activities to something produced ; he becomes conscious of the work experience. We assume that this new dimension has been acquired as soon as we observe in the child the systematic effort to produce a new entity. Our observations have enabled us to set up definite criteria for distinguishing between the behaviour of the child whose activities with material express a striving toward production from that of the child whose central urge is the practice of function irrespective of the material with which he is occupied. This differentiation leads to two highly relevant and basic definitions for this phase of childhood. Play is that activity with or without materials in which bodily movement is an end in itself. We define work as the systematic effort to create a new entity. Between the second and the sixth year this constructive or work aspect comes to dominate the child's activities to a great extent. At first the child makes only a nameless something, generally with blocks. Later the child names and indicates the significance of the thing he has made. Since the child at this stage names his products regardless of what

PLATE IV

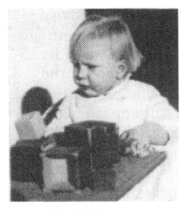

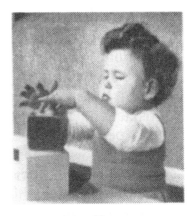

12

13

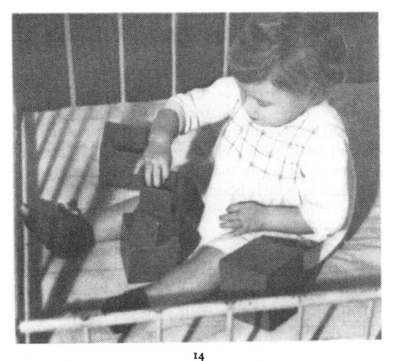

14

12. Boy 1 ; 6 puts Blocks one on the other.
13. Boy 2 ; 0 puts Blocks as well on as into the other.
14. Girl 1 ; 9 makes a Tower of Blocks.

[*face p.* 82

they look like, we consider this kind of work naming, symbolic. Later, from about 5 years on, the child's aim becomes the realistic reproduction of a definite object. A normal child of 5 or 6 has, as a rule, learned to set realistic reproduction as the goal of his handling of material. It is obvious that this transition from activity that is primarily concerned with the establishment of movement patterns, to activity that utilizes these patterns only as a means to a constructive end is of far-reaching significance. Let us imagine two children. One is walking back and forth, pulling a toy train ; the other is building a bridge out of blocks. What is the essential difference between these two forms of activity ? The first child can stop and start his activity whenever he likes ; it involves no goal. The second child has set himself a task, that is, his activity ends only when the work is completed. In order to make a bridge this child has to stick to his activity until the bridge is finished. The child learns in this way to persevere until a job is done. One might ask the question : since this is only a play situation, why do we consider the completion of the task so important and necessary ? As the next chapter shows, 80 per cent of the junior school children tested who failed in the first grade did so because they had not acquired this work attitude during their play development before coming to school. This retardation is the result either of slow maturation or more frequently of a lack of play materials.

This is usually the case with children from very poor homes or institutions. We have also found that children from well-to-do families lack the work attitude because they have received too much assistance during their play from grown-ups. Our clinical findings have led us to the conclusion that school and work maturity are practically synonymous.

As we indicated previously in the description of the child's social development, this capacity to set himself a task and persevere until it is completed influences all of its responses, especially the social ones. The child who undertakes a self-imposed task will accept one from another person. The child in this stage begins to understand the concept of duty.

We have thus far established the transition from functional to productive maturity as a continuous aspect of child development that begins with approximately the second year and ends with the sixth. The question might be asked, can this be maintained with such definiteness or are not individual differences very great ? This leads to our next problem.

Two recent studies, one being prepared for publication, and having been made by the ethnologist *Adolf Bernatzik* in the Salomon Archipelago, and the other by the *Lotte Danzinger & Liselotte Frankl* in Albania,[18] have enabled us to conclude that the transition from functional to work maturity is the expression of an innate developmental trend that is characteristic for the normal child irrespective of specific environmental influences.

As previously mentioned, the Albanian children are so bandaged in their cradles during the first year that they can move neither hand nor foot. When at first unbound they are unable to hold anything and yet within a period of two hours they cover all those steps for which our children require many months and finally are able to perform the age characteristic test. The same holds good for the 2–5-year-olds. They of course are allowed to move about freely, but they have no playthings and are quite passive and lethargic. They are at first afraid of toys and are clumsy in handling them. And yet within a few hours they can almost achieve those performances that are normal for their age. This is illustrated in the following example.

Fatima, 4 ; o. There are blocks and a doll lying on the floor. F. picks up the doll and moves it. Another child calls her attention to the blocks. F. holds the doll in one hand and with the other hand she holds one block against another one. Doll is taken away. She piles several blocks on one another. Looks around ; the tower collapses ; she rebuilds it and walks away. Later she returns to the blocks ; places them alongside of each other ; holds two of them together and says : " These are the same size." Looks at experimenter ; places the blocks alongside of each other ; when asked what it is, she laughs and says : " A store." She then takes the tower between her hands, lifts it up, it collapses ; she says : " That's too bad, now it's spoiled." She then rebuilds the tower, destroys it and laughs.

At first Fatima holds the blocks together like a one-year-old. She then begins gradually to build them horizontally and vertically. Finally she gives her work a name and with that attains the normal performance for her age. The question presents itself at this point : if a child can achieve a normal development without having had previous experience, what rôle, if any, does practice play ? It is clear that a lack of practice cannot check the development of a maturing pattern that is psychobiologically determined. This does not, however, justify the conclusion that practice is unnecessary. Although the Albanian infants, freed from their swaddling clothes at one year, can sit upright, crawl and walk after a short practice period, they nevertheless carry out all these movements with much more inhibition and clumsiness than normal children. In addition, they have been deprived of all opportunities to become acquainted with those objects in their environment that the normal unhindered child can make. One might say therefore that lack of practice cannot prevent the basic psychobiologic functions from developing, but checks that free exercise of inherent abilities that is indispensable for a healthy maximum psychic development. The diffuse and indirect effect of such a defective environment is most frequently observed in institutionalized children. Such children, lacking as they do play and social opportunities, are backward not only in their reactions to people and materials but are hindered in the development of all their potentialities. *Martha Sturm* has demonstrated that the child in the family situation touches on the average 71 different objects in the course of a day, a child in an institution only 14. As a consequence the personality development even of children coming from poor families is better than that of well-cared-for institutionalized children. For every 100 children between 1 ; 3 and 1 ; 5 brought up in a family, who succeed in achieving a normal level for block building, only 33 institution children succeed.

In the second place, it can be shown that it is impossible to teach the child, regardless of the amount of practice, those tasks for which an innate disposition is not already present, and that, on the other hand, the better the instruction is adapted to a disposition that has already appeared the easier it is to teach the child.

The Albanian children, for example, were unable within the short practice period to achieve all of the tests for their age-level without assistance. They duplicated them, however, as soon as they had seen them performed. Fatima, for instance, built only in one dimension, i.e. she placed blocks either on top of, or alongside of each other. When her mother, who was very much taken with the many-coloured blocks built in two dimensions, i.e. she built simultaneously in a vertical and horizontal direction, Fatima imitated her immediately. Four-year-olds for whom two-dimensional building is not yet characteristic do not imitate after seeing it done.

Recent American investigations have brought some very interesting results in regard to maturation and practice of various activities.

Arnold Gesell and Helen Thompson [19] carried out the following experiment with a pair of female identical twins from the first to the eighteenth month. From the forty-sixth week on, that is the tenth month, twin T. was trained in climbing and in the handling of hollow blocks, for six weeks. Twin C. was prevented from getting any special training in these two fields. The main results are as follows :

I. Climbing.

(1) In the beginning T. was entirely passive and needed help. During the first sessions she climbed the steps 3–4 times within a period of 20 minutes. After 4 weeks of training, i.e. at the age of 50 weeks, she climbed the steps alone and with great enjoyment.

(2) C., at the age of 53 weeks, climbed the same steps unaided and without any previous training, in 45 seconds, 7 times during the first attempt. After 2 weeks of training at the age of 55 weeks, C. climbed the steps in 10 seconds, T. at the age of 52 weeks, after 6 weeks of training, in 26 seconds.

(3) At the age of 55 weeks C. climbed much better than T. at 52 weeks, although T. had begun training 7 weeks earlier and had trained three times as long. The advantage resulting from 3 weeks of maturation explains this difference.

(4) The behaviour pattern that the child acquires is basically determined by the developmental level at the time of training. At the end of the training period, T.'s climbing was largely crawling, whereas C. walked.

II. Hollow Blocks.

T. was trained from the forty-sixth to the fifty-second week 10 minutes daily to play with hollow blocks. At the end of the training period there was no difference in this respect between the behaviour of T. and C. who had had no special training.

Gesell's results have been partly modified as a result of a recent similar investigation of *Myrtle McGraw's*.[20] She trained one of a pair of male identical twins over a much longer period. The child showed the primitive beginnings of climbing and swimming during the first year and in the second learned to roller-skate, whereas the brother remained far behind in some of these activities ; others he failed to learn entirely. In spite of this, however, the fact that the child was unable to master certain complex movements such as tricycle riding and that he developed no more rapidly than his brother in sitting, grasping, crawling and walking in spite of intensive training indicates the limits of trainability and the dependence of intrinsic developmental factors on maturation.

A study made by *Josephine R. Hilgard*[21] demonstrates as clearly as *Gesell's* how the acquiring of skill depends on maturation. She trained children between 2 and 3 years to button, cut with a scissors, and climb a ladder. One group of 10 children were trained for 12 weeks, a control group of 10 children were trained for a week at the end of this time. It was found that the second (control) group achieved the same degree of skill in the one week of training which was given three months after the first group had begun, as the first group achieved in the 12 weeks.

The dependency of successful learning on the level of maturation is even more pronounced in the case of intellectual activities than in the case of physical ones. *Arthur Jersild* [22] trained children from 2 to 11 years of age during a period of several months in various fields ; the older ones in the recognizing of colours, free association, tests of bodily strength : the younger ones in strength of grip, rhythmic tapping and reproduction of musical intervals. Comparisons were made between these performances by groups of 121 trained and 127 untrained children, and it was found that training had a marked effect on the acquisition of physical strength and skill in singing. In so far as free association and the naming of colours was concerned, the gain was slight and of short duration. The degree of maturation and the innate capacities of the individual were much more decisive factors than the special training. In experimenting with identical twins variation in individual ability need not be considered and it is possible therefore to segregate maturation from practice acquisitions very clearly. In the *Hilgard* investigation the factor of individual ability was to a certain extent eliminated in that only those children were used for the experiment whose first performances were approximately the same. Generally speaking, the talent factor makes a clear-cut differentiation between it and the influence of training as such, difficult. All of the investigations in this field have demonstrated that training was more successful with those children whose maturation in the activity in which they were being trained was well advanced, than with those children who were just beginning the maturation period. On the other hand, it is self-evident that the maturation level for a particular activity must not be too advanced. It is important to establish as accurately as possible the most favourable time for training. This has been found to be true in regard to many physical activities as well as in learning to speak, although we have as yet not enough exact data. We will discuss this problem later in relation to the school age.

As has been already mentioned, the impulse to make something out of material is a developmental step that all normal children have made by the time they are six years old. The fact that a child has succeeded or failed in making this step is generally an indication of the extent of psychic unbalance or intellectual retardation present. *Olga Marum and Irene Jaskulski* [23] were able to show that cases of border-line feeble-mindedness could reach this level, but that in cases of feeble-mindedness they either failed entirely to reach it or barely managed to make a primitive beginning. The two cases that follow were taken from the above-mentioned study.

Gerhard (5), 5 ; 9, 2 ; o. He places one block on another until he has built a high tower and all the blocks have been used. He begins all over again when the tower collapses. He does not show much perseverance, runs around, throws the blocks on the floor.

Gunther (7), 6 ; 5, 1 ; 7. Is given building blocks ; among them is one that is shaped like a column. He lays it flat on the table and rolls it back and forth. Demolishes something he has built and throws the blocks all over the floor. Takes a tin disc away from another child and rolls it along the floor. An Easter egg is lying on the table. He stands it on one end and spins it. He sits on the floor and draws a string to which several balls of yarn have been attached, swiftly across the floor. He sees a board with two wheels in a corner. He gets it and rolls it back and forth. This brings him in the vicinity of the sewing-machine and he begins to turn the wheel back and forth. He tries to spin a slate, swings a stuffed dog around on a string ; takes a doll-carriage away from a little girl and rolls it back and forth ; gets a plate that he tries to spin like a top with both hands. He twists or spins everything, especially things that easily lend themselves to it. He is concerned mainly with twisting, rolling and swinging things. He shows also the beginning of block-building activities. He sets up a knitting-needle and places balls of yarn on it vertically. When the tower falls down, he sets it up again and repeats this four times. He places blocks one behind the other on the same plane. He shows the greatest interest for play that involves movement.

He uses material largely for this purpose and shows only slight understanding for play with blocks.

Although children use certain materials in a sequence which is determined by their development, the preference for specific materials is also to a large extent determined by individual, typological and sex factors. For instance, all children prefer materials with which they can build during the first and second year. From the fourth year on, however, only the boys prefer building materials, while the girls are interested in other materials. *Louise Farwell* [24] demonstrated this in an interesting study.

She made 300 kindergarten, first- and second-grade children, play approximately 30 minutes daily for fourteen days, with play material that they were allowed to select from 13 various materials. They were, clay, plasticine, and damp sand for modelling; drawing and painting equipment; sewing equipment both for paper and cloth, buttons, etc.; building materials of cardboard with scissors, paper nails, paper dolls, etc. The experiments were carried out in two institutions, both of which had kindergarten and first and second grades. The youngest kindergarten children were 4 ; 9 ; so that the average age of the children studied is 6, 7 and 8 years ; i.e. in part, that which we consider the pre-school age, in part, the early school age, which we will discuss later.

The results showed that a correlation between a preferred material and this age-level is only partly demonstrable ; that above all the child's sex and school experience, i.e. his familiarity with

93

certain materials and equipment were the deciding factors in establishing preferences.

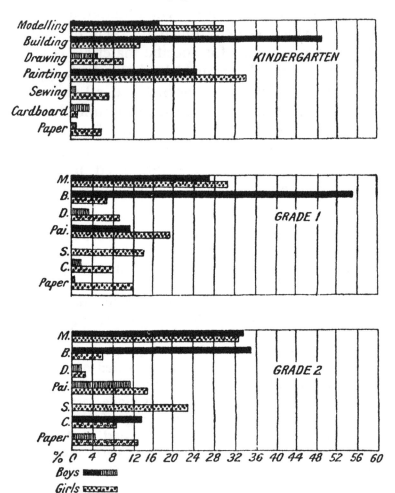

FIG. 10A.—Choice of Play Materials. (*After Farwell.*)

We see the effect of development in the increasing interest for a large variety of materials. The

94

younger the child, however, the more exclusively it devotes itself to the three favourite materials.

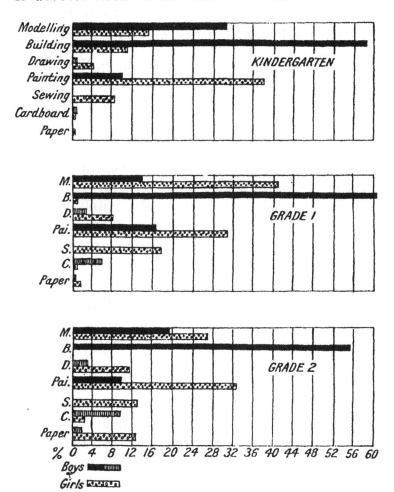

FIG. 10B.—Choice of Play Materials. (*After Farwell.*)

If we accept with *Farwell* the length of time that a child plays with a given material as an indication of preference, it becomes clear that the three materials, building blocks, modelling and painting equipment, are the three favourites, i.e. those with which the children occupy themselves most. These three materials take up 50 to 75 per cent of the total playtime of the children in all the phases, although building blocks are preferred to this extent only by the boys. The preference for blocks predominated absolutely among the boys of all phases, among the girls modelling predominated in one institution and painting in the other.

Modelling and painting take alternately second and third place among the boys.

For the girls, painting and modelling were first and second choice respectively, except that the girls of the second grade in one institution preferred sewing. Building blocks were third choice, with some fluctuations, among the youngest children ; among the older ones, sewing, drawing and paper work.

The boys without exception were uninterested in paper work and sewing. This was not true of the girls, who were interested in all the materials without exception. In one school first- and second-grade girls ignored building and cardboard work, i.e. constructive activity ; in the other school the girls in one of the grades ignored drawing.

In general, one can conclude that the boys prefer constructive materials to all others, while the girls select the more adaptive and expressive materials like paints and clay. This difference stands out as determined by the sex of the child in spite of and independent of the influence of practice, or experience, since it is clear that familiarity with various materials is possible for all the children in these institutions, irrespective of sex and degree of maturity.

Although, for both sexes, work maturity is achieved with building material, it remains the favourite only for the boys, while the girls transfer their interests to other materials in the third and fourth years.

It is a matter of common knowledge that girls do not prefer building materials and this has often been experimentally shown. *C. Philippi van Reesema* has informed me of an experiment that she has carried out that has not yet been published. She hit upon the idea of distributing paper, bits of cloth, etc., with building material. The little girls who previously had shown no interest in building began at once to make tables with cloths, beds with covers, etc., by combining the building blocks with the other materials. This experiment should be repeated with a large number of girls and boys so that the results can be definitely established.

Farwell is correct in using the duration of an activity as the measure of the child's interest and in evaluating those activities that the child pursues for the longest periods as those for which he has the greatest interest. It is important to add that sustained attention for one activity varies greatly from one individual to another. *Franz Beyrl* [25] and *Helen Shacter* [26] found that individual differences are greater in regard to the capacity for concentrated work than in regard to preference for a given material. *Beyrl* set up the following chart for four-year-olds.

TABLE IV

INDIVIDUAL DURATION SPAN OF BUILDING ACTIVITIES
OF FOUR-YEAR-OLD CHILDREN

46	Minutes.
7	,,
21	,,
21	,,
39	,,
44	,,
11	,,
26	,,
53	,,
63	,,

In order to get age or group variations one can only compare maximum or mean duration periods. If one compares the mean play periods, it becomes clear that an age increment is acquired in spite of the large individual differences.

TABLE V

MEAN PLAY PERIODS OF VIENNESE CHILDREN IN BUILDING
AND IN ASSORTING PLAY

Ages in Years	Building	Assorting
3	24 minutes	15 minutes
4	32 ,,	32 ,,
5	53 ,,	68 ,,
6	48 ,,	78 ,,

One sees in the chart that the interest of the three-year-olds was held longer by building and that of the five-year-olds was held longer by games that involved assorting. In a series of American studies the mean duration of activities was found to vary considerably and all were shorter than those of our children. This is partly caused by the selection of inadequate tasks.

In *Shacter's* study large individual differences in the sustained attention of pre-school children were confirmed. She presented to boys and girls, 3, 4, and 5 years old, attractive play materials such as multicoloured blocks, pictures and pegs. Some of them had to be sorted, others had to be arranged in a specific pattern. The sustained attention of the individual children for the specific age-level activities showed large variations. The deviation

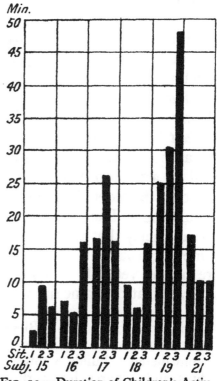

FIG. 11.—Duration of Children's Activity with Play Material. (*After Shacter.*) Playtime of subjects 15–21, using three materials.

99

of the three-year-old girls' attention was between 4 and 34 minutes, for the five-year-olds from 5 to 29 minutes. The same is true for the boys, who in addition showed less capacity for sustained attention than the girls.

The fact that some aspects of the activities with materials are determined by age, others by sex and others by individual differences is of great psychological importance. Recent studies made by *Hans Volkelt* [27] and others by *Hildegard Hetzer* [28] contribute something to this problem. *Volkelt* had children build with coloured blocks. It was found that the younger children, 2 to 5 years, paid no attention whatsoever to the colours, and that only the older children made use of the colours in building. The protocols of the smaller children reveal clearly that their aim is exclusively to build something that will remain standing, but that they are not as yet able to take the colours into consideration at the same time. An example follows :

Hellfried H. (2 ; 10). Block box 1, red-blue. H. takes out the 12 blocks, 6 red ones, 6 blue ones, immediately ; builds a tower, puts his hands on his hips and admires his work. " It is still standing ; hasn't tumbled down yet." Then, his facial expression tense, he pulled quite slowly at one of the bottom blocks until the tower collapsed. When it crashed he laughed delightedly at the noise, collected the blocks and began all over again. This was repeated several times. In building a tower he alternated in his selection of colours, but this seemed to be accidental since the alternation was not regular.

Another time he began by building a railroad; then suddenly changed his mind and began to build a tower.

Hellfried is obviously still fascinated by the tower and surprised that it remains standing, i.e. that he has actually succeeded in building something. He is so completely preoccupied with this fact that he cannot pay much attention to the colours. On the other hand, the four-year-olds already show an occasional interest in colours. An example follows :

Elfriede G. (4 ; 3) at first laid out a square of coloured discs without taking the various colours into consideration. She then placed five red half-cylinders alongside of each other and then began a second row of green ones. Since there were only four green cylinders available she was unable to make the two rows even, and asked : " Do you have another one like this ? " and completed the green row with a red cylinder ; thought it over for a while and then said, " Or I can take two away " and then took two red half-cylinders away. There remained one row of four red cylinders and another of four green ones. There was present in this design which was laid out rather than built, a definite preoccupation with colour arrangement.

Hildegard Hetzer in a recent unpublished study of the use of colours in drawing, got exactly the same results. The small child discovers the colour dimension in the handling of materials very gradually, not because it cannot enjoy colours as well as the older child, but because it cannot as yet spare enough attention to isolate this dimension.

Once colour has been discovered as a quality of materials, as a general developmental acquisition, its application varies with the individual. *Volkelt* found that the 4–6-year-olds prefer the multi- to the solid-coloured materials in 9 out of 10 cases. The 7–10-year-olds in 3 out of 10 cases, and the 11–13-year-olds in 4 out of 10 cases, showed no interest in multicoloured materials. These changes are in all probability determined by age-level. In addition, *Volkelt* describes the following individual tendencies :

(*a*) The symmetrical and asymmetrical use of colours by children who take cognizance of them.

(*b*) The realistic or non-realistic use of colours, although the non-realistic application of colours is characteristic largely for the 4–6-year-olds.

(*c*) Building in a given style disregarding a definite representation, which *Volkelt* calls " Sachsinnfrei " (without meaning). He claims that after a time he can distinguish by its style the building of the various children from one another. Individual differences are so great that a line of demarcation could not be found between the building of boys and girls. Unfortunately that which distinguishes one type of building from another was not further described.

Research in this field up to the present has brought us the following general conclusions :

It would seem that an advance in any given

direction is at first largely determined by general developmental trends and that individual variations appear when the child attempts to utilize the recently acquired increment ; for example, all children build at first and then later draw and paint.   Later on the boys are especially interested in building; the girls, however, transfer their interest to drawing and painting.   All children at some time or other discover that materials either have colour or do not ; later on they single out some specific material ; representation is at first symbolic for all children and later realistic ; but symbolic representation remains the most adequate for certain individuals.   We will go into this problem in greater detail in one of the following chapters.

CHAPTER VI

THE PSYCHOLOGICAL SIGNIFICANCE OF ACTIVITY WITH MATERIAL FOR THE CHILD

WE have already learned that the main characteristic steps in the development of the small child's activities with materials are : (1) The transition from the unspecific to the specific handling of materials. (2) The transition from the manipulation to the forming of material. This second step must be examined more closely. What is it that the child produces ?

We found that the child piled up blocks vertically, piled up sand and poured it into forms, and made all sorts of things out of plasticine, such as balls, rings, and crude reproductions of animals.

What differentiates this handicraft of the six-year-old from that of the ten-year-old ? The ten-year-old, for instance, is interested in working with the radio and all sorts of electrical apparatus. His goal is a practical one ; whereas the younger child's work with plasticine, sand or blocks has no such purpose. One would, however, expect that a child whose main aim is to produce something would, for instance, in working with plasticine or clay, try to make a pot or some other usable object. The pre-school child's failure to do this is not primarily due to an inability to manipulate suitable materials, but rather to the fact that it has not yet reached a point where it is at all concerned with practical goals. It is remarkable that the developmental path leading to the production of useful forms out of material should be so long and circuitous.

Although the child is surrounded from birth by countless articles that are put to daily use, and although the child in grasping for its bottle at the age of 6 months and in learning to feed itself with a spoon at one year, makes use of various objects in one way or another, it does not hit upon the idea of making something for its own use. Strangely enough, the young child prefers to make a symbolic rather than a real, practical object. The pre-school child instead of making a usable cup makes a form which it calls a cup. This is a representational rather than a practical act. For the child, at least in civilized society, it is characteristic that its first creative efforts are largely intellectual and that only later does it create in a practical, utilitarian sense. Since the child's productive activities pass through an ideal stage before they reach the real, practical level, it will be necessary at this point to turn our attention to this aspect of the psychic life of the pre-school child and compare it with that of the school child.

What does this representational interest mean to the child ? As we shall see, until about the eighth year the child expresses only partially or not at all the need to make something useful ; it is exclusively interested in representing things. What is responsible for this impulse ? A comparison between the children of primitive and civilized peoples shows that the children of the latter participate very eagerly in play with materials. *Danzinger and Frankl,*[29] in their study of Albanian children, found that they were not in the least interested in making practical articles. In a recent expedition to the Salomon Islands, *Adolf Bernatzik,* in co-operation with the Vienna Institute, collected material regarding the psychological development of the children of some very primitive tribes. His complete findings are being prepared for publication ; for the present he has sent me the following information. The children, at a very early age, help with the cooking, wood-chopping, fishing and hunting, and occasionally even devote themselves entirely to securing a living. Play with materials takes place only during those months when there is no hunting and fishing and then it is very similar to our children's plays. In general, it can be said, that the more the child is drawn into the sphere of practical adult activity, the less its play life develops.

Tradition certainly plays a large part in directing the activities of children of civilized peoples towards play with materials. It is to be expected that the extent to which children play in this way is dependent upon the amount of free time and materials which they have at their disposal. Children who begin to work quite young are inhibited by a lack of time. *Bernatzik* found that the amount of time that primitive children spend in play is determined by the severity of the struggle for existence, which varies from tribe to tribe, since the grown-ups must call upon the children for help if living conditions are difficult. The same holds for the children of civilized peoples.

It becomes clear, therefore, that those children who are not required to perform actual labour, concern themselves to a large extent with the creation of representational rather than of practical objects. It is only gradually that the child begins to express a desire to make a box that can be used or to construct a radio or knit a jumper. What, then, is the psychological significance of representational construction? What do we mean by representation?

Karl Bühler,[30] in his studies on language, has designated the naming of objects as the representational function of speech. He distinguishes this function in human speech from that of the expressing of emotion and that of influencing others. The representational function establishes a constant connection between signs and objects. Once the child comprehends the naming of things, it has grasped the essential principle that this constant connection between signs and objects is of practical significance. Herein lies its first speech experiences. It learns that one can be placed on a stool if one calls out " 'tool ". Although the pre-school child learns names in its mother tongue in relation to definite objects, it is nevertheless clear from its behaviour that he believes such names can be applied to any object at random. It has been observed that at a certain period in every child's life it gives names ad libitum and inconsistently to its own movements and to the forms that it makes out of materials. The child here tries to extend the application of the naming relationship and so discovers a new world, the world of the imagination and of symbols. Once the child of a year or so achieves the level of imaginative experience, all of its activities are coloured by it. The child makes a movement of some kind, later it does something with materials, scribbles some marks on a sheet of paper and calls them a steamship, and attributes to the drawing those characteristics that a ship has in reality, such as movement, etc. Something can be made out of some material other than that actually necessary to make the real object. This substitute material stands for the real material, since it has been named after it and it is possible in this way to make any number of things very easily that in reality could never be made. According to *Karl Bühler's* [31] theory it is the characteristic of the intellect that it enables functions to be exercised in a way and on materials other than those corre-

sponding to reality. Without incurring any practical responsibilities the child can try to make
things in the course of its play. One has called
these play patterns in which the child, by imitating
certain activities, attempts to create the illusion of
a real activity or object, fiction play. The naming
of these activities and objects we consider a symbolic one. All of the representational play of
the small child, with the exception of its purely
manipulative activities, is fictive and symbolic,
and is outgrown approximately at the beginning
of the school age. The transition can be best
studied from the development of the naming of
objects that the child makes. At first the child
in manipulating a material investigates its nature
and possibilities and in the process forms something. The next step is made when the child
gives a name to something it has made after it is
completed. The following protocols of this phase
are taken from a study made by *Bergemann-
Könitzer* [32] on work of children with clay.

Ruth, 4 ; 11, rides up and down and around with
a piece of clay, makes believe it is a steamer. Peter,
4 ; 5, who has been rolling clay, imitates her and makes
" puff and shh . . ." sounds.

Herman, 3 ; 10, attaches a piece of clay to a wooden
stick and calls it a hammer ; places it on the window-
sill. Hans, 5 ; 4, makes clay cubes and attaches them
to a stick ; he calls his work a " Birthday spread ".

Fritz, 4 ; 11, is delighted with something he has
formed accidentally. The teacher asks him what it
is. He thinks for a while, then answers, " A jumping-

jack." Hellmut, 5 ; 0, finishes his first piece of work, brings it to the teacher and points to it in great excitement : " A . . . sort of . . ." (Gunther mixes in and says, " A pigeon ".) Hellmut : " Of course, that's what it is, a pigeon."

Step by step the naming function develops. For a while, a thing is named while being made, and finally before the work is started. This pre-arranged name exerts no influence on the form produced. As early as the 4–5 year, however, a purely symbolic designation is replaced by a more realistic one that eventually leads to the realistic productions of the school child. Of this, more later.

The following age-levels should be kept in mind : the two-year-olds begin to designate their activities by name ; the three-year-olds name the things they build during and partly before the work is begun ; the three-year-olds as yet make no attempt to draw realistically. Representation of any kind develops much more slowly in play with constructive materials, mechanical toys like the " Meccano ".

It is at this point necessary to determine the significance of representational production for the child. We will have to look for accurately described reports in order to get a picture of the facts as they are. A few examples taken from *Eugenie Hanfmann* [33] follow :

Horsti, 3 ; 5, after finishing a task : " Look at that. I can make that too ; I can make everything."

Mariechen, 5 ; 3, " I can make that too. I can make a railroad and everything."

Leander, 3 ; 8, talking to himself while building : " Who can do this ? I can."

When Mariechen, 5 ; 4, for example, placed two different-coloured arch blocks together, looked at it in astonishment and cried out joyously, " It's a real ball with corners, and when you put it down, it stands."

From *Otto Krautter* [34] :

Another form that is discovered shortly after the sphere are the hollow impressions that are made by pressing the fingers into a soft mass. R. tried this with a small piece and cried out joyously : " A little pot, a little pot." She finished it by adding a long piece on the side for a handle.

Then H. presses a clay ball into a thin sheet. He bends in the edges because the border was irregular, flattens it out again and produces a cup form. When asked what it was, he answered, " That's a ship," and then, " No, I won't know what it is until it's finished." Finally he makes something that resembles a key. He explains, " One uses this to put a cake into the oven. I'm making a cake now ; later it will have to be baked."

From *Bergemann-Könitzer* :

He then begins to make a locomotive and at the same time talks to Hellmut about other things. He tries repeatedly to fasten the wheels that are made out of thin layers on to the body of the locomotive, but is so nervous and impatient that they do not hold. In order to keep him from spoiling the work and aggravating himself, I help him attach the wheels. Now he begins to sing : " I am making, am making, am making a fire engine with a ladder and a hose and a pump." (This is repeated in a sing-song several times, then fast, like a story.) " I saw a fire in the city by the . . . bridge." (Insistently, almost threateningly to Hellmut.) " When it sprinkles it will run you over if you don't get out of the way."

The following moments are clearly brought out in these protocols :

(1) The child is happy and proud that he has succeeded in making and completing something.

(2) The act of making something stimulates a lively flow of ideas and images. This series of ideas and images as we know from observing children who are listening to fairy tales is especially fascinating for the child of pre-school age.

(3) The child establishes with the help of those things that it has produced, its first contact with the world of the grown-ups. Such a relationship to the real world the pre-school child achieves only in a fictive, imaginative, symbolic sense, which becomes realistic at the school age.

The making of something out of material enables the child to experience the awareness of his own effectiveness and ability that constitutes the pleasure of creating. Representational production awakens for the child the world of ideas, fantasies, imaginings and introduces him to the things and events in the world and life around him. The child of this age has no interest in making something that is actually or really usable. This is the school-child's goal. Naturally the representational world that the pre-school child creates is limited and schematic. Even at this age, however, one comes across an occasional child whose work is highly individual and varied.

Four-and-a-half-year-old Gunther, for example, described above by *Bergemann-Könitzer*, produced during a period of several weeks (the exact time was unfortunately not given), 85 different objects out of clay ; during the same period the next best performance among the other children was 42 and the average was 12–15. Not only the number but also the variety of forms produced by Gunther was very unusual. It was clear from his devotion to modelling that his interest for this sort of activity was much greater than average, but also that he needed it profoundly. This is an excellent example of an individual creative drive that seeks to express itself with this material.

A consideration of Gunther's case leads us to the problem of talent, and its expression ; one of the most important problems that comes up in the discussion of personality. We find a four-year-old who shows a passionate interest in modelling, who manipulates the material much more efficiently than the average child and whose work is strongly coloured by emotion. This characterized his work with clay almost from the very beginning, as soon as he had made a few unspecific forms.

Bergemann-Könitzer also found that there were marked differences of style for instance between Gunther's and Peter's modelling, who was the next best in point of variety and number of forms produced. Gunther worked with large masses and was interested in concrete forms. Peter rolled the clay into thin rods and used them to outline various forms, frequently abstract ones, such as a pentagon, etc. He paid great attention to details, modelled the finger-nails and counted accurately, whereas Gunther attacked large problems. He was also very critical of his own work ; P., on the other hand, made telling criticisms of the other children's efforts, but was quite satisfied with his own. The phenomenon of criticism and self-criticism as a general developmental and individual characteristic we will take up later.

The function of representation like that of form production is acquired in the course of normal child development. Representation is intimately bound up with intellectual development, and although it appears for the first time in connection with speech it is carried over to other kinds of activity. It is to be expected therefore that this function will be absent when we are dealing with extreme cases of feeble-mindedness, and that the absence of the function of representation is a sign of unquestionable feeble-mindedness. We are not surprised therefore to find in the previously mentioned study of feeble-mindedness of *O. Marum*, that the under-development of this function is always present.

Two four-year-olds are given as examples, who cannot name anything at all, and eight- and five-year-olds who name their product only when asked to ; a nine-year-old who names his product only after he has begun to form it. A large number of the children acquire this function as late as the sixth to the sixteenth year.

Representational production enables the child to express himself. Pride and joy at completing something, the transference of fantasies to a material, the establishing of a bond with the life of the adult ; these needs are satisfied by the exercise of this function. As we shall see later, the realistic production of the school-child serves an entirely different group of needs.

THE SCHOOL AGE

CHAPTER VII

THE SCHOOL BEGINNER

WE already know that at about the sixth year the child reaches work maturity, which means that from this age on the child handles any material that it happens to lay its hands on constructively. As we have indicated this step has important consequences for the child's entire development. The following example should make clear the difference between the activities of the small child and the child that has reached work maturity.

The mother of two boys of 3½ and 7 years had just taken down the washing. She placed the clothes-pegs in a basket on a chair near the table in the kitchen. The boys gathered all the clothes-pegs together and filled their aprons with them. The elder boy, kneeling on the sofa, placed all of his clothes-pegs on the table, and made a horse by putting several of them together. While working he was silent, and when he was finished he clapped his hands with joy and asked me triumphantly if I knew what it was that he had made. I answered, " A horse." He was pleased that

I had recognized what he had built and then took the clothes-pegs apart again. He began to build again and there followed consecutively a house, an aeroplane, and a motor-car. As he finished making each object he asked me to identify it. He always tried to put as many clothes-pegs as possible into each construction.

The younger brother had at the same time arranged his clothes-pegs in two cardboard boxes and fastened the boxes to his wagon. While the older brother was building he rode around several times in the kitchen, then stopped at the sofa near his brother and said : " Good day, I am the baker. Do you need anything ? " The older boy answered : " Yes, give me twenty rolls." The younger boy thereupon gave him some clothes-pegs out of his boxes and said : " That costs 20 pfennigs." The older brother then pretended that he was counting out money into his brother's hand and laid the purchased clothes-pegs on the sofa. He did not, however, use them in his building, but considered them rolls. The younger boy rode around several times, even going into the hall. He then sold rolls to his brother again.

While the seven-year-old boy uses the clothes-pegs for building, the small three-year-old plays a game of pretence with them. The older one constructs something, the younger one gives the clothes-pegs a fictitious character and uses them to represent rolls. He can start and finish his game whenever he likes ; the construction, on the other hand, is a task which must be brought to a conclusion. The child in constructing something out of materials learns to accept and complete a task. Most of the five-year-old's play is constructive in character. The child understands this play activity as work. A five-year-old boy was heard sighing while making a building out of blocks. When asked by his mother to interrupt his game for a time, he said : " No, I have to finish my work." He has set himself a task and wants to finish it.

The wilfulness and laxness of the 2–4-year-old is replaced to a certain extent by the serious attitude of the 5–8-year-old. He is ready to work, i.e. to accept and complete the task which is given to him.

This is the foundation and major prerequisite for successful school adaptation. An analysis of the work in the first grades of the Viennese elementary schools has demonstrated that 80 per cent of the first-grade children who fail, do so because they have not yet developed the work attitude in their games before entering school.

Lotte Danzinger [35] conducted this study with the aid of a group of teachers. It was found that only 6 per cent of the failures are in one subject ; 50 per cent are in two, and 44 per cent are in three. This means that failure in the first grade is seldom due to the child's inability to perform successfully in a given subject. There are, of course, individual cases of reading disability, for instance, but they are rare. Failures in the first grade are due, as a rule, not to special disabilities, but to a general disability that is manifested whenever the child attempts to perform anything. The causes may be many and varied.

The child may simply be retarded because of a slow rate of maturation, for which he makes up later. In other cases, and they are very frequent, the school difficulties are not the result of retarded maturation but of environmental factors. It is possible that a child who is given no materials to work with, may as a result be mentally retarded. This happens frequently with children who are brought up in institutions. Institutions as a rule maintain a very high standard of hygiene, but are rather backward psychologically and pedagogically. Children from well-to-do homes give the impression in the first grade of being especially bright largely in consequence of their having been provided with constructive play materials.

Danzinger, in her investigation, found that the majority of the children who had difficulty in finishing a task were unusually passive. This passivity was as a rule associated with marked physical weakness, under-nourishment or bad health. Good health and sufficient nutrition are indispensable if the school beginner is to achieve the willingness and ability to overcome those difficulties that every task presents. Sickly and under-nourished children show from the very beginning of their school careers that they cannot meet requirements ; they are passive and lack the energy necessary for the carrying out of their class work.

Danzinger's findings are in accord with other investigators in Vienna, America, Germany, and

Russia. They have without exception found a high correlation between mental and physical capacities, especially for the younger children.

The data that follows seems to contradict one psychological theory, namely, *Alfred Adler's* [36] theory of compensation for physical inferiority by intellectual success. It happens frequently that adults who are weak and delicate physically are capable of high-grade intellectual performance. *Alfred Adler* built his theory on this fact of compensation ; the theory, namely, that individuals who are physically inferior in some respect make every effort to compensate by achieving extraordinary success in some other direction. *Adler* assumes that this compensatory drive functions from early childhood on. What can our investigations with children contribute to this problem ?

We know, first of all, from our tests that in early childhood there is always a correlation between good physical and mental development. It is true that there are children who although clumsy with their bodies or hands show excellent speech development, and vice versa, but we never find decided physical weakness associated with good performances of any kind in early childhood.

The same holds good unquestionably for the early school years. *Paul Lazarsfeld* [37] analysed material gathered in a study of several thousand Viennese school children and came to the following result : In the first, second and third classes good school work correlates positively with good physical development ; in the fourth and fifth classes two large groups appear, the type of child whose physical and mental development are in harmony with each other, and those who show a correlation between bad physical development and especially good school work.   In other words, the younger the child the greater the dependence of its school performance on physical well-being. The ability to compensate, that is, to achieve intellectual success independent of physical health, appears around the ninth year.

Our finding, in so far as the lower grades are concerned, were confirmed by a study directed by the Russian, *Netschajeff*.[38]   He tested 4-8-year-olds and found that their school work improved with an improvement in nutrition, and vice versa. *Netschajeff* compared three groups of children, one well nourished, the second not so well nourished, and the third on the verge of starvation, in three tests. The degree of retardation was found to be in direct proportion to the degree of under-nourishment.

Several German and American investigations have found a definite positive correlation for the higher grades between good school work and good physical development.

Else Liefmann [39] studied primary school girls who averaged ten years of age. Those who had been left back averaged eleven years, and were neither as well developed nor as well nourished as the average. She found further, a high correlation between talent and good physical development as well as size and weight. *Liefmann's* results are essentially the same as *Leta Hollingworth's*.[40] She studied a group of highly gifted children between nine and eleven years of age, with various tests, in regard to weight, size and strength. In comparing them with children of average and poor intellectual performance a consistent positive correlation between intellectual performance and physical development was found. The thirty-five most intelligent children are in every respect the best developed physically. They excel the norm set up by *Bird Baldwin* for unusually well-developed children. The weight coefficient for children whose I.Q. is under 65, between 90–110 and over 135 is distributed as follows :

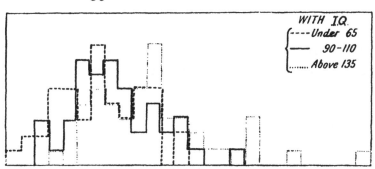

WITH I.Q.
┌---- Under 65
┤ —— 90–110
└........ Above 135

FIG. 12.—Weight-height of 9–11-year-old Children.
(*After Hollingworth.*)

The gifted children are also superior as far as general health is concerned. *Hollingworth* reports a study of high-school students made by *Sandwich*,[41] who selected the forty best and forty poorest students and tested them for physical defects. The results were as follows :

TABLE VI

CORRELATION OF PERFORMANCE AND PHYSICAL DEFECTS IN SECONDARY SCHOOL STUDENTS

	The 40 Best	The 40 Poorest
Number of physical defects . .	27	*125*
Average number of physical defect per student	0·71	*3·41*
Percentage of students without defects .	52·5	0·00

These results would seem definitely to refute the compensation theory as a fundamental psychic mechanism and are surprisingly similar to ours.

It is certain that successful mental as well as physical performance are primarily dependent on those drives that are the product of good physical condition. In other words, strength in the purely physical sense seems to be the first and most basic prerequisite for good mental performance. There exist undoubtedly in addition other tendencies such as ambition, compensation for inferiorities, etc., that are not connected with the physical condition. It would seem, however, that second-ary drives of this nature are not fully at work in the young child, especially since he is as yet incapable of self-criticism.

The child finds everything that it has made itself beautiful, more beautiful than that made by anyone else, and it develops a capacity for self-criticism only very gradually. Just as the two-year-old points with pride at something that he has built successfully the child in the kindergarten and lower grades still is lost in admiration of his own work.

Self-praise and criticism of others, as we know from several studies, are primary attitudes that appear as soon as the child begins to evaluate what it does as performance.

When we ask ourselves how these attitudes, which we can illustrate with examples and which the idealistic educator will find very unwelcome, can be explained, we must bear the following facts in mind.

From the first year on we find negative response and effect present whenever the child is unable to master a given situation, positive response and effect when it succeeds. This tendency is also at work in the situation mentioned above. The devaluation of the performance of a rival apparently enables the child in some way to maintain a sense of its own worth and seems to confirm the importance of its own work.

Studies of self-criticism and the criticism of others during the kindergarten-age have been made by *Ovide Decroly*, *Pearl Greenberg* and *Hildegard Hetzer*.[41a]

Ovide Decroly, assisted by Mlle *Degand*, made a large collection of the spontaneous, self-praise, self-criticism and the criticism of others expressed by children from 4 to 13 years of age. Numerous examples show (1) that there is a primary tendency in the direction of self-praise under any and all circumstances, that is, regardless of whether the actual facts are taken into consideration or not, and whether the success is the result of capable performance or of accident.

> Raymond, 6 years and 6 months, for example, by accident put his foot into a hole that had been formed by an iron bar and cried out triumphantly : " None of the others can do this ; I'm the only one who knows how to do this."

(2) A child takes every opportunity to compare itself with other children who are either being praised or criticized, who complete a task successfully, or who possess something. For example :

> Fr., 4 years 6 months, was praised for the very clean shoes that he was wearing. M., 5 years, said at once, " I also have shoes, and I've even got a velvet dress."

(3) There is a primary tendency to deprecate the other child.

> P., 9 ; o, notices that Henry has forgotten to bring her school book. Turning to the teacher she says : " Naturally Henry has forgotten to bring my book again ; he's always that way."

(4) In those cases where a child fails to solve a problem, the problem is depreciated as unimportant.

> Jy., 10 ; 6, is criticized for his poor handwriting and answers : " Oh well, a nice handwriting is dumb, anyway."

Only from the eighth year on do children begin to assume an appreciating attitude toward other children. This has been substantiated by two experimental studies which showed also that the younger child strives constantly to heighten its own importance at the expense of others. Only later does it begin to show a capacity for recognizing the efforts of other children.

Pearl Greenberg,[42] in a research " Competition in Children " made in Vienna, gave children of 2–7 years competitive building problems and studied : (1) Those remarks made by the child spontaneously about his own work and the work of others ; (2) the opinion of his own work and the work of others which the child expressed when asked " Whose is prettier ? "

She found that : (1) the 2–5-year-olds rarely expressed spontaneous opinions. If they were expressed at all they were always positive for their own, negative for the work of the other children. Spontaneous negative self-criticism makes its first appearance at 6–7 years in 10 per cent of the cases in comparison with 70 per cent of self-praise ; 4·5 per cent of the opinions of the 5–6-year-olds are spontaneous positive criticism of others. The judgments passed when asked directly, " Whose is prettier ? " tend to lean somewhat in the direction of the work of the other child. Sixty per cent of the 2–3-year-olds do not understand the question. Insecurity in passing opinions also occurs occasionally among the older children. In approximately 3–4 to 4–5 of the cases favourable opinions of their own work, and in 1–4 to 1–5 of the cases favourable opinions of the work of others were passed. There is no essential difference in this respect between the two- and the seven-year-old children. Favourable criticism was always made of the work of the older children, frequently older brothers or sisters, never of the younger ones. The wish to degrade the other is expressed frequently, when not directly, indirectly.

> Example : The observer says to B. 4 ; 6 pointing out to him a house that B. 3 ; 11 has built, " Isn't that pretty ? " B. 4 ; 6 : " Yes, but he hit me with a stone once." Or G. 4 ; 6 says about B. 4 ; 6, " He can't do anything. I can build a railroad."

In like manner, *A. L. Emmons* [42a] in studying dexterity (manual skill) in young children finds absolutely no correlation between the degree of development of self-assertion and the degree of dexterity. The self-consciousness of young children is completely independent of their objective performance. *Emmons*, as well as the author just mentioned, does find a correlation between the ability to criticize oneself and the age of the child. A correlation between self-criticism and degree of intelligence is also substantiated, in that the more intelligent child is capable of self-criticism at an earlier age.

Hildegard Hetzer and *Hanna Winkowski* [43] came to the same results in their study, *Criticism in the Kindergarten*.

Twelve children out of seventy-three in two kindergartens were observed for six days in regard to critical and self-critical remarks. The ages ranged from 2 ; 11 to 4 ; 6 years.

Fourteen cases of self-criticism were found to ninety of criticism of others. Only eleven out of the ninety were favourable opinions and only sixteen criticisms of the older children were made, almost all of them unfavourable. From the very beginning there are occasional objective criticisms, but as a rule they are subjective, whether favourable or not.

Example : Harry, 3 ; 6, says enthusiastically to Elfriede, 4 ; 9, " Isn't my tower high ? " E. sees that H.'s tower is higher than her own and answers, trying to avoid the issue, " Mine is prettier ; yours isn't pretty."

Favourable opinion. Anna, 3 ; 9, to Peter, 3 ; 8, " You haven't said good morning to me yet." Peter makes a deep bow and says good morning. A. answers, " Peter, you've never bowed as nicely as this to me before."

M. E. Smith,[43a] as well, finds many more negative criticisms made by pre-school children than positive ones.

Hildegard Hetzer with Edith Podelil[43b] made a study of criticism and self-criticism in the school age. They observed 6–9-year-old girls in the first three grades. Three to five girls out of approximately forty showed a tendency to criticize the others a great deal and were as a consequence disliked. In the first two classes, criticism is made of appearance, possessions and performance. In the third grade the teacher and the school work is criticized in addition. Self-criticism is as yet mainly favourable. They observed objective self-criticism in the third grade, and in one case, underestimation of own work.

Objective self-criticism makes its first appearance at nine years of age and, as we shall see later, it initiates a new psychic development that can be described as the transition to realism on all levels. It is only then that the child is able to see its own work as it really is.

As has already been mentioned, the success or failure of the child at the beginning of its school career is not dependent entirely on the possession or lack of ability, but largely on the child's capacity to understand and accept work responsibility as such. The 4–5-year-old child usually has the intellectual equipment necessary for the understanding of school work in the first grades. As a consequence, misguided adults teach 4–5-year-olds to read, write and memorize quotations. The child of school age has achieved that which the 4–5-year-old lacks, namely, sufficient maturity to enable it to assume work responsibility. This maturation is dependent on the development of will and personality. The most rapid intellectual advances are made between the second and fourth years. From the fourth to the eighth year this development takes place at a much slower rate. The difference between the mental world of the 6–8-year-old and that of the 4–6-year-old is not very great. There is simply a steadier and more serious attitude towards the tasks it is given. The extreme individual variations of the pre-school age disappear. From the many studies that measure intellectual advance we have selected the following as an illustration. *Kathe Spiegel* studied in Vienna the development of verbal memory in children between two and five years by letting them repeat words and verses. The following table gives us a clear picture of the slowing down of the learning process :

TABLE VII
PROGRESS IN THE LEARNING OF WORDS AND VERSES

Age in Years	Percentage Learnt of 90 Syllables		Percentage Learnt of 35 Sentences	
	Boys	Girls	Boys	Girls
2	12·3	10·0	14·0	11·0
3	33·0	33·0	37·2	36·9
4	63·0	64·5	67·5	69·5
5	73·5	80·0	73·0	82·0

The greatest learning advances are made from two to three and three to four years. From then on the rate of advance slows down considerably. Also from then on the girls catch up with the boys. *Josephine C. Foster,*[44] who in a similar investigation with children from $2\frac{1}{2}$ to $4\frac{3}{4}$ years, told stories and had children memorize material, found the same rapid progress from the second to the fourth year. She found that from one to ten words were reproduced after the first reading by all the children, but that when the reading was repeated the individual performances became sharply differentiated.

TABLE VIII
PROGRESS IN LEARNING TO REPRODUCE STORIES

Number of Words Memorized after 4 Repetitions	Age in Years	Number of Words Memorized after 9 Repetitions
2–3	2	8–9
10	3	30
30	4	70

Individual differences in learning at this age are great and seem to depend on various factors. *Annette Herzmann* studied visual memory in pre-school children in order to eliminate the language factor. Chocolates were placed under variously coloured paper boxes and the child had to remember under which boxes the chocolates had been placed. In this and similar experiments 4–5-year-olds from middle-class families were from 30 to 50% more successful than children from the proletariat, for the 2–3-year-olds the difference was not so great. *C. A. Probst* [45] tested five-year-olds for general information about time, place, plants, animals, etc., and found that the two main factors in determining individual variation were individual capacity and social level. The mean figure is 81·2 for the higher social group, 63·8 for the lower; the general average is 71·6. It is significant that the extremes of individual performance range between 52 and 107 points. *Helen P. Davidson* [46] taught children between the ages of 3 and 5½ years to read. She found a higher correlation between reading and " intelligence " than between reading and chronological age, but above all a very high correlation with social level. At this level the effect of innate intelligence on the intelligence tests score cannot be generally differentiated from the effect of environment. For this reason *Gertrude P. Driscoll* [47] also comes to a negative conclusion as far as the prognostic value of the intelligence test for pre-school children is concerned. *A. Netschajeff*, [48] the Russian, also found that variations between individual performance for the younger children of the 4–8-year-old group when tested for intelligence were so great that he felt it necessary to set up a special theory to explain it.

Before the second year, the maturation level plays a seemingly greater rôle than environmental factors. *Lois C. Strayer* [49] carried out the following interesting experiment with the twins that *Arnold Gesell* studied. She taught one of the twins, at the age of 1¼ years, Spanish words for five weeks, and five weeks later subjected the other one of the twins to the same training. She found that the five weeks of maturation exerted a profound influence on the success of the learning process. The relationship between general maturation increments and individual differences can be described as follows : General maturation is of major importance from birth to the second year. From the second to the sixth year great individual differences make their appearance. We have stated the greatest individual differences between the second and fourth year. Between the sixth and the eighth year the rate of intellectual growth and of the development of individual differences slows down considerably. The greatest advance at this age, in contrast with the earlier level, is in the direction of the development of will power rather than in the direction of intellect.

As in the case of learning, the intellectual interests and psychic world of the 4–8-year-old children do not show very great fundamental individual variations. Children's intellectual interests can be determined by the questions which they ask.

Under my direction, *Margaret van Wylick* worked over the questions of a 2–4-year-old girl, collected by *Elisabeth Kawohl*,[50] and those collected by *Jean Piaget*[51] of a six-year-old boy. Both collections together made up twice 700 questions, and it was found that the majority of them for both children were concerned with cause and motive. The questions of the four-year-old were largely concentrated on names, time and place, whereas the questions that appeared for the first time at six years showed an interest in rules and in how things are made. Activities and motives are the central interests of the pre-school child and the school beginner. As we will see later, the child transfers its interests from human beings to the objective world.

The small child is not only interested in human

activities but it attributes human motives to all natural events. It personifies animals and things in that it endows them with motives, names them and understands their movements as the product of desire and will.

The name as such is of especial importance to the small child. " If there were no names, one couldn't make anything," said a child to *Piaget*. A five-year-old whom *Pyler* [51a] presented with unknown and unnamed toys in the course of an experiment said to him, " How nice it would be if they only had names " *Usnadze* [52] had 4–7-year-old children name meaningless objects and found that especially the four- and five-year-olds enjoyed it. The thing becomes personified for the child through its name ; it becomes a similar creature. In addition the child until about its eighth year thinks that things act and desire in the same manner as himself. This anthropomorphic attitude can be discerned in the first sentences that the child says at about 1 ; 3.

" The soup has a cold," says Inge B. at 2 years, 2 months, on seeing a bubble on the surface of her soup. This seemed not an analogy for her, but the description of a reality.

Or Bubi S., 3 ; 5, " The blood thought the black court-plaster was a black man [chimney-sweep] and it ran back quickly."

Or " The fly is still trying to break the window."

Or some examples from *Piaget* :

Cli, 3 ; 9, " The auto sleeps in the garage." " It doesn't come out because it is raining."

Bad, 3 ; 0, " Are the bells awake yet ? "
Nel, 2 ; 9, sees a wooden cross. " Did it cry when the hole was made ? "

A survey we made of Bubi Scupin's anthropomorphic remarks made during his first six years shows a trend similar to the studies made by *Piaget* [53] in that he also finds that at about the sixth year the child is no longer absolutely certain that things possess desires and feelings. The child begins to suspect and to look for a form of existence that differs from that of the living, feeling organism. As several examples indicate, however, it takes a long time before the child can finally free itself from the belief that all things have a psychic life of their own. The Bubi Scupin chart, which we worked out, follows :

TABLE IX

THREE TYPES OF OBJECTS OF ANTHROPOMORPHIC THINKING
THAT APPEAR IN THE COURSE OF DEVELOPMENT

	Age in Years							Calculated figures
	1 ; 6– 2 ; 6	2 ; 6– 3	3– 3 ; 6	3 ; 6– 4	4– 4 ; 6	4 ; 6– 5	5–6	
1. Group : Inanimate objects	62	42	37	31	14	—	—	26·5
2. Group : Natural phenomena	7	42	37	38	29	33	20	29·5
3. Group : Plants and animals	31	16	26	31	57	67	80	54
Sum . . .	100	100	100	100	100	100	100	—

The above development notwithstanding, the

animistic concept is not as yet entirely discarded. The following is an excerpt from *Piaget's* talks with seven- and eight-year-olds.

Vel., an 8½-year-old boy, explained, on being questioned by *Piaget*, that only animals and not things feel something when prodded, but when *Piaget* asked, " Does this bench feel anything ? "—" Yes." " Why ? " —" Because it falls to pieces." " Does the wall feel anything ? "—" No." " When it is thrown over, does it feel anything ? "—" Yes." " Why ? "—" Because it is pulled to pieces." *Piaget*, " If I tear this button off " (pointing to his vest), " would it feel it ? "— " Yes." " Why ? "—" Because the thread tears." " Does that hurt it ? "—" No, but it feels that it is being torn."

A discussion with Kent, 7½ years old :
" If one sticks this pebble, would it feel it ? "— " No." " Why ? "—" Because it is hard." " If one put it into the fire would it feel it ? "—" Yes." " Why ? "—" Because it would get burned." " Does it feel the cold ? "—" Yes." " Does a ship feel that it is on the water ? "—" Yes." " Why ? "—" Because it is heavy. It feels the weight of the people who are on it pressing from the inside."

One sees that the child becomes uncertain, that his opinions waver. The school child no longer believes that things actually have feeling, but it cannot as yet conceive that a thing which is subjected to an attack does not feel it, just as it would itself. The concept that things act and feel persists until late in the school age.

The extent to which these anthropomorphic interpretations actually govern the thinking of the child has often been discussed. The objection has been raised that in *their behaviour toward reality* children often show the same expectation of mechanical causes and results as do adults. " As a matter of fact, the child would be very much frightened ", according to *Karl Bühler*,[53a] " if the doll suddenly started to walk or to cry " (p. 172). The child actually is frightened, as we know from an experiment with a mechanically moved doll. When it has overcome the fright it begins, in the second year of life, to do just exactly what an adult would do, namely, to examine the mechanism (*William Menaker*).[53b] *Susan Isaacs* [53c] finds in her observation material that " many disparate types of behaviour (are) co-existing in the same children, and ranging freely between the (anthropomorphic) phenomena characterized by *Piaget* to clear logical statement and reasonable action " (p. 97). How is this contradiction to be explained ? *S. Isaacs* believes that the child comprehends logically those things with which it has had practical experience and which belong to its sphere of interest ; and that, on the other hand, anthropomorphic thinking reigns in the spheres where the child has had no personal experience. We would formulate the same idea in these words : Action in practice and theoretical thinking about events are in the beginning quite disparate phenomena. Only gradually is thinking influenced by experience. We see the gradual progress in the table of anthropomorphic expressions, which narrow down to fewer and fewer objects.

The school maturity of the 5–6-year-old is, as we said above, not so much established by intellectual progress of this age but by the new acquired ability and willingness to undertake and carry out tasks. This willingness has another important consequence which is equally a symptom of, and necessary for, school maturity. The child learns, namely, to accommodate itself to a group. The pre-school child is neither willing nor able to make this type of adaptation. It prefers to play alone, with one or two other children, or it attaches itself to a favourite grown-up. It does not as yet participate in group activities, either because it is afraid of large numbers of people or because its impulsiveness and lack of perseverance result in withdrawal from the group.

Wislitzky and Hetzer,[53d] in a study of the spontaneous grouping of kindergarten children, found that the pre-school children prefer either isolation or participation in a group of two. It is significant that even in Russia where every possible attempt is made to encourage and stimulate group life, not much success is achieved with kindergarten children, who, like all children at this age, prefer to play with one companion or alone (*Krasusky*).

From about the fifth year on the child undergoes a complete metamorphosis in this respect. He participates willingly in the activities of the group. *Hildegard Hetzer* [54] in a study of street games found that the majority of the participants in games that called for large groups ranged from five to eleven years of age. It is characteristic for the games played during this age span that they follow traditional rules and ceremonies that must be strictly adhered to. Verses are sung or prescribed movements are carried out in the course of which all the children either do the same thing or different prescribed rôles are distributed. The game must be carried out as if it were a task which serves to unite the still loosely organized group.

Even in the first school classes the child who prefers to be alone is the exception rather than the rule. *Karl Reininger,* [55] assisted by a group of teachers and psychologists in Vienna, studied the behaviour of school new-comers during their first social contacts over a period of weeks. It was found that after three days of school attendance, 99 per cent of the children had established contact with one or more of their classmates. Whereas the isolation of children of kindergarten age is quite common, it becomes a symptom of abnormal, neurotic development for the six-year-old. Shyness frequently interferes with the direct expression of a wish for companionship.

It becomes clear from the very beginning that various personality types can be distinguished from their social behaviour. Some are leaders, children who display at once sufficient initiative and talent to make suggestions and to attract followers. Some are helpers, children who look for other children whom they can help and lend things to. Some are maternal, that is, they single out and take care of their weaker and more helpless neighbours. Some are despotic and tyrannize over the others. The most characteristic child for the youngest school group is the much-loved favourite ; usually a kind, gentle, charming child who makes little effort to establish contact with the others, but who, nevertheless, is the recipient of all kinds of attention from them. Then there are children who joke and make fun of others, who are constantly showing off ; and finally, there are the solitary children, the social failures. Children who are defective physically, dirty, or very poorly dressed are often ostracized by their comrades in the elementary classes. Adherence to the group at this age-level is motivated largely by the wish not to be left alone, to be one of the group.

CHAPTER VIII

THE NINTH TO THE THIRTEENTH
YEAR OF LIFE

PARENTS, teachers, and all those who have to do with children know that during certain periods they can be easily directed and taught and that during others it is very difficult. It is, for instance, a matter of common knowledge that the child between the second and the fourth year is especially difficult to handle. It is easily upset, and often impossible to control. We have already taken up some of the problems connected with this phase in Chapter IV. The 5–10-year-old presents relatively the fewest difficulties. Whereas every three-year-old behaves like a " problem child ", the problem child between five and ten years is an exception, and, as a general rule, neurotic. An insight into the extent of problems of upbringing for the various age-levels can be gained from the age distribution of the children brought to a child guidance bureau that was run in connection with the Vienna Clearing House for Children.

TABLE X

AGE DISTRIBUTION OF THE CASES BROUGHT TO THE CHILD
GUIDANCE BUREAU

Age in Years	Percentage of Cases
0– 2	11
2– 4	24
4– 6	20
6– 8	15
8–10	7
10–12	11
12–14	12
	100

One can see from this that the highest percentage of problems occur between the second and the fourth year. Cases of obstinacy present the greatest difficulties for parent and teacher. These difficulties then decrease steadily until the tenth year. From then on there is another rise which culminates between the fourteenth and sixteenth years. The period of least difficulty lies between the eighth and twelfth years. This conclusion, which we have established statistically, has been confirmed by *Erich Benjamin*,[56] one of the leading child psychotherapists, who found that the 8–11-year-olds make up the smallest percentage of his patients.

If we can ascertain which factors are responsible for the balance and freedom from conflict that characterize this age-level, we may be able to shed some light on the transition that occurs at the end of this period.

One of the most outstanding and significant

characteristics of the phase from eight to twelve is that it marks a culmination in the development of physical strength and vitality. *Frieda Sack,*[57] in a very detailed study, made a survey of all the available data on health, disease, mortality, morbidity, etc., and found that there is no other period during which the mortality rate is as low or the resistance to disease as high as during the tenth year. The child himself is usually conscious of his own strength at this age. A ten-year-old boy writes in his autobiography, " I am strong and vigorous. I stand straight, my arms and legs are strong." And a ten-year-old girl : " I am very brave ; I like to do things that require courage."

Adolf Busemann [58] found in studying a collection of autobiographies that the mentioning of the body reaches a high point between the ninth and tenth year. *Hildegard Hetzer,*[59] in a study of the distribution of boasting for different age-groups, found that the 8–12-year-olds contributed the highest percentage. Especially for the boys of this age, boasts about strength form a part of their normal talk. We know also from the work of *Karl Reininger* [60] that the leader at this age is generally selected because of his strength, skill in football or some other sport. The child who dislikes sport, who lacks courage, or is sensitive, has a more difficult time with his companions at this period than at any other.

Physical development and skill at sport become

so important for the boy of this age that it often occupies the centre of his interests and activities. *E. A. Menaker, Frieda Sack,* and *Lotte Danzinger* [61] carried out an extensive study in Vienna of the ages at which the various sport activities begin, and of the significance of and preference for different sports at various age levels.

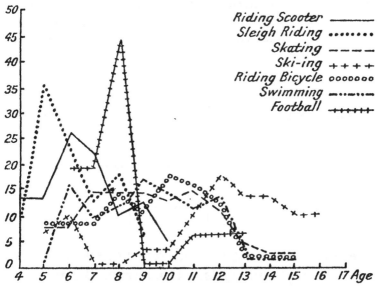

FIG. 13.—Average Age for the Beginning of Various Sport Activities (from four to sixteen years).

They collected, in addition, American, German and Swedish statistics regarding the development of sport performance and the earliest age at which sport records are made. Many sports are learned in early childhood. It was clear, however, both from the material that was gathered and from conversations with, and direct observation of children, that the main source of enjoyment for children up to eight or nine years in sport was the free expression of movement, which we call functioning, rather than the achievement of a given level of performance. The child makes superfluous movements just for the fun of it. In the ninth or tenth year the child's mobility begins to concentrate on effective movements ; he wants to do a sport well. Therefore we find a considerable decrease in the variety of movements.

TABLE XI

DISTRIBUTION OF THE VARIETY OF MOVEMENTS BETWEEN THE AGES OF 6 AND 12

Ages	6–7	7–8	8–9	9–10	10–11	11–12	Totals
Boys . . .	20·00	20·40	20·00	20·00	10·85	8·45	99·70
Girls . . .	14·70	22·90	21·10	16·50	16·50	8·25	99·95

There is as yet no great difference in sport ability between boys and girls. Only from the twelfth year on do major differences make their appearance. The average performance of the boys improves steadily up to the eighteenth year, while the girls' average steadily decreases from the fourteenth year on to the seventeenth. This physical differentiation that begins with about the thirteenth year will be discussed in detail later on.

The impulse towards intensive training and the

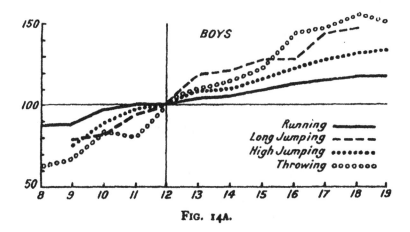

FIG. 14A.

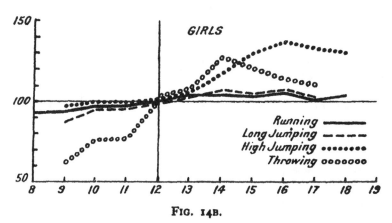

FIG. 14B.

FIG. 14A and B.—Average Progression in the Performances of Boys and Girls.

ambition to make record performances does not generally make its appearance before the sixteenth year. Several adolescents said : " One must start a sport at ten, but one cannot make a record before seventeen."

TABLE XII

MINIMUM AGE FOR RECORD PERFORMANCES IN TRACK ATHLETICS

Track Activity	List of the 30 Best Athletes		Olympic Candidates		German Committee for Physical Training
	Men	Women	Men	Women	Men
100-m. Dash .	19	17	20	20	22
200-m. Dash .	21	18			
Long-distance run					
5,000 m. .	22	18	21	19	22·7
10,000 m. .		(800 m.)		(800 m.)	
100-m. Hurdle	20	18	21	—	—
		(80 m.)			
400-m. Hurdle	—	—	—	—	—
Broad Jump .	20	18	21	19	—
High Jump .	20	16	23	18	22·4
Pole Vault .	21	—	23	—	—
Spear Throw .	19	18	24	19	23·7
Shot Put . .	20	18	24	17	—
Discus Throw	21	17	28	19	—
Hammer Throw	22	—	—	—	—
Ball Throw .	—	18	—	—	—

FROM NINE TO THIRTEEN

E. A. Menaker collected the data of physicians who had devoted much study to sport regarding the most favourable time for athletic training and earliest record performances.

TABLE XIII

AGES MOST SUITED FOR BEGINNING ATHLETIC TRAINING AND RECORD PERFORMANCES ACCORDING TO THE STATEMENTS OF SPORT PHYSICIANS

Kind of Sport Activity	Age	Author	Remarks
Applicable for all branches of sport	18	W. Schnell	Overtaxing the growing organism and heart.
	18	F. Gaisbock	
	18	K. Pauluzzi	
	18–20	J. Müller	Tests of endurance are only for the mature individual with a normal heart.
	18	W. G. Losert	
Track :			
Dash . . .	19	H. Altrock	Competitive sport should not begin sooner.
Long-distance run	20	R. Ackermann	Too great a strain on the still-growing organism.
Marathon . .	22	O. Hug	
800 m. . .	20	K. Worringen	
200 m. . .	18	K. Worringen	
Other Sports :			
Swimming. .	17	J. Müller	Should begin with short distances.
	19	H. Altrock	Strain on body and heart.
Rowing . .	17	J. Müller	
	18	K. Worringen	
Bicycling . .	16	J. Müller	A strong spine and heart are essential.
Skiing . . .	17–20	H. Rautman	
	18–20	H. Altrock	

Thus the group from eight to twelve, which is now under discussion, is not as yet interested in record performance but in skills and in group play. It is for this reason that boys of this age prefer football and girls basketball or " Völkerball ". Some of the boys say : " I enjoy playing in a group," or " Football is great, because one has an opponent."

This brings us to the second characteristic feature of this phase, namely the social factor, which is of great importance for this age. The group begins to play a dominant rôle in the child's life. Ostracism from the group is a bitter experience for the child of this age, although a few years later solitude is preferred. The 8–12-year-old wants to be a member of the group, to participate in its activities and never to be alone. The wish to be alone is almost invariably even more neurotic for the child of this age than for the 5–8-year-old. Children of this age enjoy the organization of, as well as participation in group life. Clubs and other organizations are founded, whose rules, or laws, require the performance of certain duties and responsibilities. In this way the child is given valuable training and preparation for future social and civic duties. Group games are preferred to all others during this period. Skill in social and competitive games is also emphasized. From the tenth year on those games begin to be preferred that are played without strict adherence to rules and where an individual leader can develop.

This wave of physical development, with its interest in sport and physical strength, introduces an element of conflict into the school situation, since it is directly opposed to the increasing intellectual demands and responsibilities that the school now begins to make. It is, however, counterbalanced by an equally strong mental acceleration. It has been demonstrated in a large number of studies that from nine to eleven there is a sudden forward spurt in memory, logical, abstract and critical thinking. We found in agreement with the researches of *Piaget* mentioned above that the 8–10-year-old emancipates himself from the anthropomorphic point of view, begins to look for, and understand cause and effect relationship and moves rapidly towards a realistic conception of the world. The following example illustrates this transition :

A six-year-old boy explains to a friend why the magnet with which they are playing attracts iron. He says : " You know, the magnet has a soul and tiny little hands, so tiny that we cannot see them, and it is with them that he pulls the iron towards himself." This is an anthropomorphic interpretation, that is, the magnet is personified. The child presumes that the magnet has a soul, will, human motives and functions with invisible organs. Up to about the age of five, the child thinks that every object is endowed with an intelligence and will like its own. After the fifth year the child's belief in this anthropomorphic interpretation of natural phenomena begins to weaken. He casts about for other explanations and often comes close to the correct one. A nine-year-old girl, for instance, when asked where dreams come from, answers : " Our thoughts do not sleep, they go on while we sleep, so that we can watch them and know what is going on in our minds." It is clear from these attempts to explain the world around him, that the child of this age needs an introduction to logical, scientific thinking in order to proceed with its intellectual development. The 8–12-year-old is realistic ; he wants to find out what things really are and how they function.

This all-embracing intellectual curiosity is a basic factor in the development of the child at this age. At no other time can the school rely so largely on the child's willingness to learn even by rote. A skilful teacher can get better results in this age than in any other, especially when by incorporating a game or competitive element into the learning situation.

The chart that follows was taken from an exhaustive investigation of " The Growth of the Memory Function ", made by *E. Brunswik, L. Goldscheider and E. Pilek*,[62] and shows that the first peak in the development of memory is reached by about thirteen years.

The powerful intellectual interests of this phase alter the attitude towards school work in many respects. The beginner, i.e. the pupil in the first three elementary classes, is willing and able to master the problems that are given him. But the child of 8–12 is eager and ambitious out of interest in his own work. This new attitude towards school work is expressed after the ninth year by the development of the child's own intellectual interests, a much greater degree of absorbed participation and a sense of responsibility. *Elsa Köhler and Ingeborg Hamberg,*[63] describe in a very thorough study the development of interest

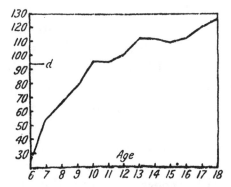

FIG. 15.—Development of Memory for Boys and Girls together from 6 to 18 years.

in the study of German in a Swedish school class. They found that the playful enthusiasm of the ten-year-old in learning a new language is replaced by the serious interest and will to learn of the twelve-year-old.

In a study, " The Ability to Learn Independently ", *Albin Hermann* [64] found that the fourteen-year-old children were so dependable that there was a very slight difference between the learning success of a group that was left entirely to its own resources and one that was controlled by a teacher. The good students did better work when left to themselves ; only the average and poor students were more successful when directed. It was also found that students of this age were not satisfied simply to solve a problem in a routine manner, but that they developed original methods with which the surest, most reliable results could be obtained. *Elsa Köhler* [65] in a similar study found that a self-reliant serious attitude toward work was characteristic for the 11–14-year-old child.

It is clear from the foregoing that we can expect that the 5–6-year-old is mature enough to comprehend the nature of a task and to carry it to a successful conclusion. If this is not the case, a retardation is present. In order to consolidate this work attitude for children from the sixth to the eleventh year, considerable help from the teacher is still necessary. On the other hand, from the eleventh year on the acceptance of independent work responsibility is not only spontaneous and natural but is more common than the play attitude. An interest in intellectual work makes its appearance around the ninth or tenth year and after the eleventh year special intellectual concerns begin to develop.

With the first appearance of endogenous interests and increasing intellectual enterprise and maturity, performance and success assume an entirely different significance than for the school beginner. Objective criticism and a sense of responsibility also develop. Several interesting studies have been made of this phase. *Clara Helwing* [66] gave children, seven to thirteen years of age, mental problems, in such a way that mistakes were suggested but could be self-corrected later. She found that in the course of the two years between seven and nine, satisfaction with their own performances as contrasted with self-criticism, dropped from 70 to 40 per cent.

Hildegard Hetzer investigated the favourable and unfavourable criticism made by children of their own paintings, and found that the unfavourable criticisms made up 55 per cent of the total and increased steadily from the ninth year on. From the tenth year on 60 per cent of the children were capable of preponderantly objective self-criticism. This attitude differs fundamentally from the self-satisfaction of the small child and school beginner as described in the preceding chapter. The school report also begins to play an important rôle at this age and is intimately related to the new objective attitude and standard of performance that the child now achieves.

Hildegard Hetzer [67] in an investigation of great practical value attempted to find out the general effect and significance of the school report for the pupil. She found that the 9–13-year-olds more than any of the other children, accepted the school report as an adequate evaluation of their own work. The 6–8-year-olds expect a good report unconditionally. The wish is still father to the thought as far as their work is concerned. Children of this age make no attempt to determine the objective correctness of the decision that they find in the report ; the fairness or unfairness of the teacher's opinion is as yet of no importance. The question of the fairness of the report, on the other hand, is as important for 40 per cent of the 9–13-year-olds as objective self-criticism. From the fourteenth year on, however, the adolescents reject the school report entirely as a dependable measure of their work.

H. Hetzer investigated further (1) the extent to which pupils of various age-levels concerned themselves with their reports, (2) the favourable and unfavourable effect of success and failure.

She found that boys are less dependent on the faculty opinion than the girls and that in general about one-half of the pupils were profoundly influenced by their reports. It is significant in this connection that improvement in work was affected to the same degree by either a good or bad report, whereas failure in work was always increased by a bad report. In other words, failure affects school work adversely.

Hetzer's examples prove again that the depressing effect of failure and stimulating effect of success are basic psychologic phenomena in spite of the fact that there are great individual variations. *Kurt Lewin* [68] showed this before in an experimental study with grown-up persons in a test situation where the outcome was immaterial in order to determine the effect of success or failure on the individual's own standard of performance as well as the manner in which the individual expressed emotion and criticism. Only 15 per cent of the subjects were unaffected either by success or failure, and the effect of failure is practically always negative, not at all stimulating. It is already clear at this point that the self-imposed requirements and the quality of the performance release an emotional recoil that affects the character of the work drive. This self-imposed standard and qualitative goal that makes its appearance at the very latest from that age-level on where objective criticism of his own work and a serious work attitude begins, imposes a tremendous emotional burden on the school child which can vary greatly from one individual to another, but is as a rule quite considerable.

The seriousness with which the school child, especially from the ninth to the thirteenth year, takes his school work, is expressed not only in the impression that the school report makes at this time, but also by the wish for a fair teacher. *Martin Keilhacker* [69] collected the opinions of several thousand school children regarding this matter and found that the most frequently expressed wish was for a fair teacher. This is especially true for the middle years (9–13); the younger children, on the other hand, prefer the mild, easy-going teacher and expect that this attitude on the part of the teacher will enable them to get a passing mark even when the work is not up to par. The eleven-year-olds, as a rule, no longer expect this sort of favouritism, and are therefore all the more concerned with getting a fair teacher. In describing the effect of unfairness on the part of the teacher the children say : " One loses all desire to study," or " One becomes discouraged and begins to hate everything."

The question that we have raised at this point of the emotional burden imposed on the child by the school and the retroactive effect of self-imposed standards and degrees of success on the work drive, has not as yet been systematically studied. It would be possible to find much valuable material related to this problem in the investigations of the pediatric psychotherapists like *Boenheim* or *Benjamin*, but it would be necessary to analyse their findings from our point of view. *Benjamin* [70] made a statistical study of several hundred cases in order to determine what percentage of the neurotic children and adolescents brought to the physician were unsuccessful in their school work. For the boys, he found that 50 per cent of the 6–7-year-old patients, over 60 per cent of the 8–11-year-olds and over 70 per cent of the 12–15-year-olds did poor work ; for the girls the percentages are much lower, fluctuating between 25 and 45 per cent. *Benjamin* assumes that the etiology of the girls' neuroses is more complicated and difficult to determine than the boys', for whom the burden of school failure seems to be an important factor in the establishing of neuroses. It is clear, therefore, that under certain circumstances the school can impose emotional burdens that lower intellectual receptivity.

In discussing the school beginner, we found that the success or failure with which he performed his tasks was determined by general maturity and physical conditions ; special abilities and disabilities were at this level of almost no importance. This state of affairs undergoes a radical change at about the ninth to eleventh year, as the school begins to make increasing demands and the child's own intellectual growth makes (in about the ninth year) a sudden spurt forward. We can anticipate that individual differences will become more marked as a result of this intellectual growth and this has been confirmed by a statistical comparison of performances. From this point on individual differences become clearer in all directions : in regard to interest, industriousness, and other work drives as well as in regard to special abilities. This brings us to the question of innate abilities and their development.

Two expressions are used in everyday language to describe innate, natural inherited abilities : people speak of talent and of intelligence. In popular usage they are never clearly distinguished from one another. Talent is the more inclusive concept. One designates as talented an individual who possesses a special technical or artistic ability, but under certain circumstances one describes an individual with unusual intellectual gifts as talented. Generally speaking, when we say that a child is very talented, we mean that it is intelligent, but the same expression might mean that the child has artistic abilities. When one speaks of talent one means specific inherited abilities. By intelligence one understands only those abilities that are based on intellectual processes and memory.[71]

According to popular opinion there is no question that such a thing as general intelligence exists. *William Stern*, in defining intelligence as " the general ability of an individual to consciously direct his thinking towards the solution of new problems, that is the ability to make an adaptation to new life conditions and problems ",[72] has found a formula in this direction. It is assumed then that (1) there is such a thing as " general " intellectual ability which is responsible for the intelligent performance of the most varied tasks, (2) intelligent conduct is the successful mastery of a new situation. This general intelligence or ability is differentiated from talent or special ability.

This popular assumption that intelligent conduct is built up on a substratum of general abilities has precipitated a sharp controversy in the literature. In Germany, *Wilhelm Peters* [73] has made a penetrating and sweeping criticism of *Stern's* theory. A decisive debate on this question took place between *Charles Spearman* and *Edward Thorndike*. Whereas *Thorndike* [74] denies the existence of general abilities of any kind that condition practical conduct, *Spearman*,[75] after a critical review of all the facts to be considered, concludes that there is a so-called " general factor ". He arrives at this general factor not through theoretical generalizations, but practically, as a result of correlations and statistical evidence. The correlation of various performances as well as the statistical working out of the correlated data, led to the conclusion that in the case of special abilities two factors which must be sharply differentiated are at work : (1) A general factor, *g*, which varies from individual to individual, but remains constant when correlated with specific abilities in the same individual ; (2) a special factor, *s*, which not only varies from one individual to the other but also from one ability to the other for the same individual. *Spearman* considers factor *g* universal, i.e. a basic function or groups of functions which all forms of intellectual activity have in common, although the content of this function or functions has not as yet been determined.

We can consider this factor as indirectly established and as advanced in order to explain the phenomena under consideration. *Spearman* says, " it may or may not be so that we find reasons from which we can deduce that *g* operates in such a way as to produce that which we call adequate intelligence."

Although *Spearman's* study is invaluable in that it attempts to establish objectively an intelligence factor as well as general intelligence, we cannot overlook a difficulty which *Spearman's* concept creates.* *Spearman's* definition of the *g* factor can also be applied to the

---

* Other important criticisms have been made by *Cyril Burt*,[75a] who considers a third, the " group " factor, as the essential, and by *Godfrey Thomson*,[75b] who assumes more complicated factors.

maturation factor. Maturation is a factor that varies from one individual to another and remains constant for the single performances of one individual that are correlated with each other. *Spearman's g* factor can therefore be either intelligence or maturation, that is, the intellectual performances of two individuals can vary not only because their intelligence differs but also because their levels of maturity differ. We can go even further. If as *Peters* assumes intellectual performances are intimately bound up with temperamental traits, for instance, if all of an individual's practical activities are affected by a strong emotionality, it would then be necessary to assume a third general factor from which intelligence would be diacritically isolated, a character factor which also *Spearman* assumes. These difficulties arise because one can only measure performances, never the individual as such. It is true that performance is comprehensively defined as being dependent on a factor g and a factor s. But the general factor which determines a given performance is not simply that which we usually understand as intelligence but includes also a group of moments such as industriousness, willingness, energy, etc. *Spearman* himself considers perseverance and oscillation as general. Factor g is thus much more than intelligence as such. It includes all of those moments that place the totality of an individual's mental activities on a definite level. It seems to me that this general factor is best characterized in this way.

It would be of great practical and theoretical importance if the individual moments that are contained in factor g, and that in their aggregate determine the level of mental performance, could be isolated and could present their effects independent of each other. This has, at the present time, only been accomplished in regard to a partial factor, the factor namely of age, that is, of maturation. It seems also partly proved for the factor of sociability.

The latter statement seems to be suggested by all our test work in which we find on the one hand a certain type of feeble-mindedness correlated with high sociability, and on the other hand in many cases of neurosis high intelligence correlated with anti-social tendencies. It is also confirmed by a recent study of *J. B. Russell*,[75c] who made records of intellectuality in correlation with other qualities and found sociability to be not at all correlated with intellectual capacities.

Two statements of fundamental importance regarding the partial factor age have been established on the basis of concrete investigations :

(*a*) With increasing age, i.e. maturation, quality of performance becomes increasingly independent of the age-level.

(*b*) As age advances still further, talent is differentiated, that is, the factor *g* becomes less effective than factor *s*.

In support of statement (*a*), investigations made by *Karl Marbe and Ludwig Sell*[76] offer confirmatory evidence. These authors showed that in the case of primary school children, the exclusive influence of age on performance can be demonstrated, that is, when the pupils in each class are divided up into the three groups, oldest, middle and youngest, their reports as well as their marks in individual subjects bear a clear relationship to their respective age-levels. In each of the seven grades of several primary schools the oldest children of a grade showed a consistently better average than the middle group which in turn was superior to the youngest group. Age as a factor no longer exerts such an exclusive influence in the secondary schools, although it is of importance in the upper primary school grades, though not to the same extent as in the lower grades. *Fritz Braun*,[77] a student of *Marbe's*, established this in a second study. *Marbe* makes environmental influences responsible for these differences. This assumption is untenable since some of the primary school children are subjected to the same environmental stimuli as the secondary school children, and this must therefore influence the character of their school work as well. It is much more probable that for the children of secondary school age, special abilities play a more decisive rôle than the general level of maturity. Talent is of more decisive importance for the secondary than for the primary school child because the secondary school children are already as a group selected for their abilities. We find, then, that maturity for the younger, and ability for the older school child is the decisive factor in determining school performance, and that at first general ability, then special ability make their appearance. This last statement is in complete agreement with *Spearman*. He himself bases his contention on the extensive tests made by

Cyril Burt,[78] according to whose results the correlation between a general mental test and school work undergoes the following changes :

TABLE XIV

CORRELATIONS OF THINKING-TESTS WITH SCHOOL
PERFORMANCE (ACCORDING TO BURT)

Age . .	10–11	11–12	12–13	13–14 Years
Correlations	78	81	64	59

The correlation, which is very high up to the twelfth year, declines rapidly from then on. In other words, at about the thirteenth year special abilities and general intelligence begin to evolve into separate entities. According to *Spearman*, the influence of the factor *g* on the individual's performance declines steadily from the twelfth year on and the influence of factor *s* increases. *Lämmermann* [79] tested 11–12-year-olds in twenty-two different performances both for general intelligence and special performance. He found that at this level general ability still exerted a greater influence than special ability, that is, all the correlations of specific abilities with general intelligence are very high. Drawing ability showed the lowest correlation. This confirms our findings that the correlation between single and general performances in regard to the development of practical-artistic skills is high only until the beginning of puberty.

We find, then, that the quality of school work from the sixth to the eighth year is determined almost entirely by age, that is, by maturation level ; that from the eighth to the twelfth year general ability or intelligence is the predominating influence, and that only from about the twelfth year on do special abilities begin to play a rôle. This thesis would seem at first to contradict observations made in other fields, namely, that certain artistic and technical talents often develop unusually early. The question then arises, is it not possible that special artistic and technical abilities mature earlier than the intellectual ones. For an answer we can turn to an extensive and reliable literature. The investigations of *Seashore* together with an extension of his work carried out at the University of Iowa, are the most detailed studies of musical talent that we have.

Musical talent has always been considered the earliest to develop. *Stanton and Koerth* [80] in their most recent study have shown that it is impossible to determine the exact degree of musical ability before the tenth year, but that after the tenth year no significant changes in this direction can be expected, and that no matter how excellent the training, no fundamental advances can be achieved. This talent, then, appears early, but its level can be determined only relatively late.

Many other studies of musical ability reach conclusions similar to the above. *Valentin Haecker and Theodor Ziehen* [81] carried out a very extensive study, from which the following table, showing the earliest appearance of musical talent, is taken.

TABLE XV

THE FIRST APPEARANCE OF MUSICAL ABILITY

Sex	Very Early	Under 2	2	3	4	5	6	7	8	9	10	Years
Boys	23	18	28	30	18	37	26	15	19	16	30	Cases
Girls	21	17	18	10	13	16	12	11	12	13	20	

Adolf Nestle,[82] who investigated " Musical production in childhood ", in children from the third to the fifteenth year, found that age exerts a considerable influence on the sense of pitch and on the composing of melodies, so that the girls reached a maximum of melodic skill by the eleventh year, the boys by the twelfth year, and that at puberty there is a temporary decline. He also found that the sense of pitch is fully developed by the eighth year. *Otto Reimers*[83] found that for boys between the ages of seven and fourteen years there is still considerable advance in the development of the sense of pitch, but that as early as the seventh year they were able to repeat familiar songs from memory. *Geza Révész,*[84] one of the most outstanding workers in this field, who has undertaken an exact analysis of musical talent, found that age exerts an influence on the development of musicality during the frequently quoted years from 7 to 12. *Révész,* like *Stanton,* found that this talent was affected only very slightly by practice and technical skill. *Fritz Prager*,[85] who had children from 6 to 15 years reproduce and recognize sound, speech and song rhythms, found that the average of performance undergoes no fundamental changes after the 9–10 years. Only in speech rhythms, and that is very characteristic, is an advance between 9 and 15 years discernible ; the percentage of successful performance increases from 50 to 76 per cent. In song rhythm recognition the ten-year-olds show 64 per cent and the fifteen-year-olds only 67 per cent of correct solutions.

To summarize : Even musical ability, which is the talent recognized at the earliest age, and the one relatively least dependent on age and practice, is determined, up to the tenth year, to a certain extent by maturation. Before the tenth year the degree of musical ability cannot be ascertained with absolute certainty. Occasionally unusual talent makes its appearance quite early. Children so endowed are called " Wonder children ", an expression which in itself indicates how infrequently they occur.

The same is true for mechanical talent. *Helmut Meier and Gerhard Pfahler*[86] studied primary school children from 7 to 13 years in reference to mechanical skill and found that between the 5–7 school year, that is, between the tenth and the thirteenth year, there is hardly any advance in mechanical ability. They found, just as *Stanton* did for musical ability, that mechanical talent was definitely manifested by the tenth year, and that in almost all the cases of unusual skill members of the child's immediate family had mechanical vocations or talents ; on the other hand, in no instance were they entirely devoid of mechanical ability. They assume, therefore, that mechanical skills are inherited. This question will be taken up later. Whereas musical talent has in general been found to correlate with general ability, mechanical ability seems to be to a much greater degree specialized. In 45 per cent of all the cases it was found that there was a large gap between the grade for mechanical work and the grade for the general school studies. Theoretic technical ability develops later than practical. The talented technician should be clearly differentiated from his schoolmates from the fifth school year on. *Pfahler* is of the opinion that his problems can be used as tests for technical ability by the seventh to the eighth year, that is, as early as it is possible to distinguish absence of mechanical ability from its possession. We have here, therefore, even on the level of average talent, a relatively clear and early specification.

As we know from a study, " Concerning the Development of Mechanical Talent ", made by *Vinzenz Neubauer*,[87] this technical ability is mainly a male talent ; girls achieve only at puberty performance levels that the boys have already mastered by eight years.

Drawing, like musical and mechanical talent,

169

is also frequently observed quite early. It is at this point, however, that we can question the prognostic importance of such early skills. None of the highly talented children that were discovered by *Kerschensteiner, Levinstein, Kik,*[88] developed later in such a way as to justify the expectations that their performance had aroused. When we keep in mind the astonishing fact that a large percentage of all boys are interested in mechanical things and that they occupy themselves successfully with various handicrafts and that many children paint and draw so well that they seem to give promise of great talent, but that as adults these same children are suddenly incapable of drawing the simplest object and seem to have lost all interest in mechanical activities, it becomes clear that what appears to be special talent is in reality nothing of the kind. The foregoing material would instead seem to lead us to the following conclusion :

Striking performance of any kind in childhood is an expression of general mental alertness and initiative rather than of special talent in a given direction. The gifted eight-year-old draws because drawing is the most adequate expression for this age ; at ten he will in all probability interest himself in handicrafts ; during puberty he will compose music or write poetry, and as a three- or five-year-old he will concern himself with fiction games. It is rather infrequent for really specific talents to function so early. What really happens is that a general mental activity seeks out a material that is suited to a given age-level and does very well with it. One can say that as far as the child's development is concerned this is fortunate, since in those few cases in which there was no question of a genuine talent which had led the child to neglect other fields, the child's development was unfavourably affected. For example, Anna, a child who was observed by *Elsa Köhler*,[89] had great language ability, was manually very clumsy, so clumsy in fact that it is hard to imagine any degree of successful life adaptation unless steps were taken to curb this tendency. The development of all so-called " Wonder children " is endangered at exactly this point and would lead us to expect an unfavourable future.[90]

Aside from this more or less pedagogic aspect of this problem, the fact that in general the early artistic talents of the child have no specific significance, has one important consequence for our understanding of the aesthetic experience in the life of the child. It is a remarkable fact that all children build, draw, model, sing, that is, they concern themselves with all kinds of artistic activity. It would seem to me that on the basis of the above-mentioned studies that reveal the special significance of artistic activities, we can make the following assumption : with the exception of those children who are so talented that art interests give promise of filling out the biggest part of their lives, art plays the rôle, in the development of the individual child, of an un-specific preparatory mental training. Whereas the practical productive activities of the school child remain an important part of the rest of the child's life, the child's artistic productivity is an expression of mental liveliness, and in general a non-specific expression for the individual. An intensive interest in drawing can signify (*a*) that the child possesses unusual talent which is not very frequent, (*b*) that the child is mentally alert and capable of development and is for the present applying his initiative to artistic representation.

We have found that the production of things that have a practical use begins to replace and eliminate the representation of things, i.e. artistic activity. From the ninth to the thirteenth year the child is mainly interested in technical problems and work. Many boys of this age develop their technical potentialities to such a point that they do all the necessary electrical repairs at home. But even those children who do not achieve this degree of skill are interested in all sorts of activi-ties with materials. One of the favourite occu-pations for children of this age is the collecting and hoarding of all kinds of materials. The 8–12-year-old seems to face all materials with the ques-tion : " What can I collect that is usable, that I can make something out of ? " This tendency to collect has been studied by several investigators. *Mary Whitley,*[91] *H. C. Lehmann* and *P. A. Witty,*[92] recently *Durost,* questioned altogether about 10,000 children and adolescents between 8 and 20 years about their collecting interests. Eight to thirteen was found to be the most characteristic age-group for this activity. A Viennese study of several hundred school children from 7 to 14 years made by *Lotte Danzinger* [93] showed that 100 per cent of the 11–12-year-old boys and 91 per cent of the 11–12-year-old girls collected something. Between 7 and 14 years the per-centage of boys who collect is never less than 84 and that of girls never less than 78.

The same lowest percentage of 87 was found by *M. Whitley*, but in the American studies, 10 is the age of the maximum interest. The studies were made differently, in so far as in some of them items were named, while in others the chil-dren had to name the items themselves. This causes some differences in the number of items and in the number of collections which the children claim to have made. *Mary Whitley* gives the following table of objects which children and adolescents collected.

TABLE XVI

OBJECTS COLLECTED

Pieces of string	Little ornaments
Pieces of cloth	Little toys
Rubber bands	Pieces of ribbon
Pieces of metal	Marbles
Small boxes	Small pictures
Tinfoil	Beads
Buttons	Pieces of trimmings

TABLE XVI (*continued*)

OBJECTS COLLECTED

Autographs	Letters received
Puzzle questions	Coins
Samples school work	Poems
Photographs	Prizes from packages
Funny papers	Stones, pebbles, rocks
Coupons	Shells
Stamps	Animal parts
Doll furniture	Leaves
Drawings, sketches,	Pressed flowers
Old magazines	Bottle-tops
Theatre programmes	Spools
Pennants	Paper dolls
Athletic trophies	Lists of names
Badges	Keys
Score cards	Party favours

An attempt to interpret the above findings reveals that the objective value of the objects cannot be of major importance. Stamps, books and drawings are practically the only objects that belong in this category. One might also include coupons, that can be redeemed for various useful articles in this group. Sometimes children think that their collections of shells or stones will be some day of objective value. All the other things collected, such as postcard portraits of famous football players and actors, or theatre programmes, can have only a subjective value. In most cases the mere pleasure of hoarding such materials as string, metal, boxes, which can be used for manipulation, must be the motivation at work.

When we ask the children themselves why they

collect things we get various answers. Some reply (especially the realistic-minded eleven-year-olds) that the value of the things collected is important to them ; later an interest in the objects or the pleasure of collecting is emphasized. This more or less subjective motivation is more characteristic of the girls (81 per cent) than of the boys (63 per cent). *Danzinger* found that collected objects were not only arranged and sorted, but also that objects were traded. All authors find that more than one collection is made at a time. Fifty to 100 per cent of the boys (only 28–46 per cent of the girls) repeatedly exchanged the objects that they collected. By trading, the children were enabled to experience the pleasure of new possessions. The boys of 11 and 12 years were not at all shy or ashamed to admit that they sought an advantage in trading whenever possible, and were proud of their shrewdness. Most of the collectors possess more than one collection, the Viennese children on an average of 2–4 per individual, the American children even 7–8. The orderly arrangement of collections also is an important activity. Here, again, the differences between the boys and girls are interesting.

It seems that the boys collect more systematically than the girls. The contents of the collections vary in the different age groups and both sexes. I worked out from *M. Whitley's* material the three favourite items of boys and girls in different ages. The list is the following.

TABLE XVII

THE THREE FAVOURITE ITEMS

Boys

Age	First Item	Second Item	Third Item
7	Marbles	Coupons	Magazines
8	Marbles	School work	Coupons
9	Marbles	Coupons	Funny papers
10	Coupons	Marbles	Stamps
11	Coupons	Marbles	Stamps
12	Coupons	Marbles	Coins
13	Coupons	Coins	Stamps
14	Coins	Coupons	Marbles
15	Coupons	Coins	Stamps
16	Coupons	School work	Photos
17	Letters received	Photos	Theatre programmes
18	Theatre programmes	Letters received	Photos

Girls

Age	First Item	Second Item	Third Item
7	Funny papers	School work	Rubber bands and small boxes
8	Paper dolls	School work	Coupons
9	School work	Paper dolls	Beads
10	Paper dolls	Coupons	Letters
11	Coupons	Letters	Beads and magazines
12	Letters	School work	Coins
13	Letters	Beads	Pictures
14	Letters	Photos	School work
15	Letters	Photos	Magazines
16	Letters	Photos	School work
17	Letters	Magazines	Pictures
18	Letters	Magazines	Pictures

It appears from this list that the difference between boys and girls is greater than that of the various ages. Marbles, coupons, coins and stamps are the favourites of the boys up to the age of 16, after which the trend of interest changes. Compared with the boys' practical interests, the girls appear much more idealistic. Samples of school work and letters, photos, magazines and pictures are their main items. Their more materialistic interests are expressed in the collecting of beads. The break of the interests in the girls is around 12 years of age, after which no more toys are collected.

The interests of the Viennese children are somewhat different. Stamps play the main rôle in their collections ; then coupons are collected by the younger ones, and books or photos by the older ones.

From these facts it seems quite clear that the collections have not much, or certainly not primarily, to do with the wish to possess things.

With that we come to an important point.

As a rule collecting is considered an expression of the desire to possess. Undoubtedly the satisfactions that are derived from the accumulation of possessions play an important rôle in the making of collections. It seems to me, however, that another moment is also involved ; the collection represents something for its possessor which varies with his wishes : for the adolescent from the thirteenth year on the collected objects have an ideal in addition to a real value. For the boys and girls of 11 and 12 years, however, the collection, aside from the actual worth attributed to it by the child, is valued as a plaything and for its usability ; that is, it is manipulated. This is clear from the frequent exchanges made by the boys.

An examination of the objects which a normal

boy of 10 carries around in his pockets reveals the extent to which collecting is determined by the interest in the manipulation of materials. *Mrs. Scupin* [94] once made a list of the objects that she found in her eight-year-old boy's pockets; they were : (1) a grey-black, sausage-shaped, twisted form with a giant knot—the handkerchief ; (2) a thick roll of string ; (3) a half-rusted pocket-knife ; (4) an empty matchbox ; (5) a piece of solder ; (6) the bulb of a flashlight ; (7) a shoe lace ; (8) a pencil ; (9) two crayons ; (10) four foreign stamps ; (11) two carpenter's nails ; (12) a steel pen ; (13) a wrinkled advertisement of *Liebig's* meat extract.

" I still need all of that ! " Hot tears as a part of the pocket's contents were confiscated.

Bubi was quite unhappy when his mother threatened to take all these things away. " I need all that," he insisted. The following episode taken from the biography of *Fritjhof Nansen* illustrates the keen interest taken by a boy of 10 in materials that he can work with.

The ten-year-old boy went to a country fair with his brother, and for this once they had money in their pockets for amusement. To the great astonishment of their parents, the boys came home loaded down with tools of all kinds. They preferred, instead of enjoying the pleasures of the fair, to buy their long-desired tools for handicraft. The parents, touched and probably also somewhat shamed, did not wish that the boys should be cheated out of the proper children's amusements at the fair because of their commendable interests, and sent them away with money again. The boys wandered once more down the long road and came home the second time loaded with tools.

We found in our studies that the interests of the 8–12-year-olds move so emphatically in the direction of the practical and every day that it would seem important to utilize it pedagogically. The adolescent shows much less interest in kitchen and house-work, wants to be alone a great deal, and for a time has a definite aversion to the humdrum daily routine. The 8–12-year-old on the other hand is flattered when asked for help or advice. It would seem advisable to take advantage of this tendency that expresses itself spontaneously at this age and to teach the children to do house-work and the little repair jobs that have to be done around the house, rather than to wait until puberty.

The enthusiastic interest that the 8–12-year-old has for these commonplace daily events can be used as a corner-stone upon which to build a spirit of friendship and comradeship. This is especially important since a few years later the adolescent tries to free himself from home influences as largely as possible.

CHAPTER IX

ADOLESCENCE

In the previous chapter the statement was made that the child's response to the educational experience from the eighth to the twelfth year was preponderantly positive, characterized by extraordinary vitality and endurance and as a rule highly successful. During the following developmental phase, i.e. 12 to 17 years, a metamorphosis from a fundamentally positive to a negative attitude takes place ; that also has a physical basis. The psychic balance of the 8–12-year-old was the product of good physical condition. The physical health and strength of the 8–12-year-old furnished the foundation for his psychic balance. Increased activity of the ductless glands and the onset of sexual maturity seem to disrupt the balance of the organism so completely that the psychic equilibrium also suffers. The manifestations of this upheaval differ for boys and girls. There is a greater similarity between the interests and activities of boys and girls between 10 and 12 than at any other period in the course of their development. On the other hand, there seems to be a greater difference in these respects between the 13–16-year-old boys and girls than at any other period. Some illustrations follow :

The mother of a 13-year-old boy appeals to our child guidance bureau for advice. She is in despair about her son. He had been obedient at home and had done good school work until quite recently. Then suddenly and without any apparent reason his attitudes changed. He became surly, ill-mannered, lost all interest in his school work, and spent most of his time playing on the streets with other lads. What is she to do with him ?

The mother of a 13-year-old girl appeals for advice to the same bureau. She says that her daughter who had been a model child and excellent scholar had suddenly let up on her school work. She redoubled her efforts in order to make up for her failures, but without success. She also neglected her piano studies, of which she formerly had been very fond. She is lazy, sits and dreams most of the day. She is impudent to her parents and she even quarrelled with her best friend. What is the mother to do with her ?

In comparing these cases one observes similarities as well as differences. In both cases social behaviour undergoes a radical change, an alienation from former friends and authorities takes place and activities that had been much enjoyed are discarded. On the other hand, whereas the girl becomes increasingly lazy and passive, the boy seems to be unloading superfluous strength and energy in his play activities. We have called this period the negative phase. For the girls it is characterized by diminished efficiency ; they become restless, unstable, generally dissatisfied, passive and lazy. Occasionally they exhibit the aggressive behaviour that is generally characteristic for the boys. In a study of girls by *Hildegard Hetzer* [95] it was found that this phase ceased with the beginning of regular menstruation. The negative phase was generally observed between the ages of 11 and 13 years in the middle European countries. The corresponding period for boys occurs about one year later, and seems to occur simultaneously with what for the majority of boys is the onset of masturbation.

As we have already stated (see Chapter IV), masturbation has been observed in the small child. The psychoanalyst, *Joseph K. Friedjung,*[96] considers the masturbation of young children an everyday, healthy occurrence. The pediatrician, *Curt Boenheim,*[97] on the other hand, after many years of clinical observation, is of the opinion that masturbation in young children is either a manifestation of precocious sexuality or of degeneracy. Whatever the case, the psychoanalysts also assume that sexuality diminishes between the fourth and tenth years. According to *Sigmund Freud* [98] infantile sexuality culminates in the third to fourth year and a new wave of sexuality begins at about the tenth year.

The general opinion is that masturbation as a widely distributed general phenomenon appears between the eleventh and fifteenth year. The distribution curves of *Magnus Hirschfeld* [99] and *Meirowsky-Neisser* [100] are very much the same.

I reproduce the latter one which assumes the peak at 15 years.

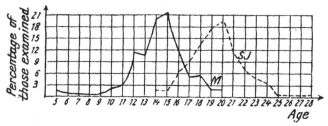

FIG. 16.—Beginning of Masturbation and Sexual Relation. (*After Meirowsky-Neisser.*)

Hirschfeld's curve reaches its acme between the twelfth and the fourteenth year, *Meirowsky's* between the fourteenth and fifteenth year. In both curves a definite ascent begins with the eleventh year. Both authors give practically the same estimate for the duration of the masturbation period. *Meirowsky* finds that for

14 per cent masturbation lasts only a short time.			
21 ,,	,,	,,	1 to 2 years
30 ,,	,,	,,	3 to 4 ,,
35 ,,	,,	,,	5 to 10 ,,

Hirschfeld considers three to four years the average duration. The general percentage of adolescents who masturbate is rated quite high. The estimates, which like the graph are based on information regarding boys, range between 70 and 99 per cent. *Oswald Schwarz* [100a] considers masturbation a normal developmental phase for puberty, but confines it to boys. There is practically no available data as far as girls are concerned. *Hirschfeld* correctly maintains that masturbation is not practised nearly as much by girls as by boys. It is much more characteristic for girls during this period to express themselves sexually in a diffuse excitability that cannot be specifically discharged and is therefore channelled off into such unspecific forms as physical and emotional restlessness, fantasies and dreams. All the data that we possess for the years of adolescence confirm this point of view. It would seem, therefore, that the fact that a fundamental difference now appears between the development of the boys and girls, whereas up to this point no fundamental differences were to be observed, should be considered the outstanding new moment of this period.

When one considers the data that we now possess it is impossible to doubt that from the first vague sexual manifestations during puberty to the more and more definite expressions in adolescence and the remainder of life, feminine sexuality has an entirely different rhythm and emphasis than the masculine. Puberty and the climacterium are the two points of vantage from which the entire development can be seen in the clearest perspective. It would seem as if sexual development follows a diametrically opposed course for the two sexes. For the woman the climacterium is a primarily physical and only secondarily psychological phenomenon, whereas to describe this period of the man's life in the same way would be medically inaccurate since one can speak of a " climacterium " here only in a psychological sense. At the beginning of puberty, feminine sexuality is much more diffuse than that of the boys. The sexual excitement that the girls experience is distributed over the entire body rather than concentrated on a specific organ which shows itself quite distinctly in the general motor restlessness of early puberty. For the boys the specific organ stimulus is of major importance from the very onset of puberty, and for this reason the tendency to masturbate is much greater than for the girls. It is more characteristic for the girl to achieve specific organ pleasure if she is awakened by another person, whereas this specificity is endogenous and primary for the boy. The rôle played by this awakening and the expectancy which it conditions in the development of feminine sexuality gives this a completely different character from that of the masculine.

It is important at this point to characterize the early steps of puberty. Two elements are present at this time for both sexes. Sexual activity has developed to a point where it achieves a complete release and orgasm by way of masturbation. As in the foregoing period, it is, however, as yet unnecessary that the actually practised or fantasied sexual function have a partner. The fantasies and wishes that are concerned with other people during this period are not sexual in the narrowest sense ; that is, the individual has a need at this period for tenderness and a desire to be with the admired person rather than for a definite sexual bond.

One can say that sexuality in this phase is still a more or less personal matter which involves only the individual's own body but not as yet a partner. On the contrary, for a while the adolescent avoids contact with his fellows and isolates himself as much as possible. In this way the adolescent passes through a period of negativism before he finds the way to a partner, especially since both sexes show a tendency during this phase to avoid each other as much as possible.

Individuals of both sexes during this transitional period show a disinclination to work until sexual maturity is reached and a certain stability is found. This fact should be taken into consideration by educators and the requirements for pupils during this phase be lowered. Quite a few cases of adolescent suicide occur during this phase. They are generally young people who have been driven to desperation by the difficulties at home and at school. Parents and teachers may often ease this desperation by a tactful explanation of the transitory character of this period. Unfortunately, however, even they seldom have a sympathetic understanding of puberty.

We observed the first drift away from school

work at the beginning of the intensive sport period. Nevertheless, the strong intellectual development that expresses itself from 10 to 12 years in an eagerness to learn and a general thirst for knowledge compensates for the drive away from study in the direction of sport. With the beginning of puberty a general restlessness sets in that diverts the youngster for a time from work. An emotional awakening that will be discussed later in detail absorbs the individual's energy. For the time being the adolescent is concerned much more with his day-dreams and fantasies which, as we know from the investigations made by *Jaensch* [101] and *Kroh* [102] of " Eidetic ", become as real as actual experiences, than with his studies. In addition, the interests of the adolescent now show a tendency towards specialization, as well as in a tendency to express themselves in part outside of school. The Russian, *Blonsky*,[103] in his study, " The Lazy Pupil ", demonstrated that so-called laziness increases with puberty and with the multiplication of the student's private interests. Students between 8 and 16 years were appraised by their teachers in regard to industriousness and laziness. He finds that (1) the percentage of " lazy " girls is much smaller than that of the boys; (2) with the exception of the second grade the boys become increasingly lazy as they get older. It is only by the time they reach the seventh grade that the girls show the same degree of laziness achieved by the boys in the first class. On investigating the problem more closely, *Blonsky* found that the increase in laziness is in direct proportion to the increase in extra curricular activities. Laziness in contradistinction to backwardness resulting from a lack of ability does not correlate positively with anaemia and sickliness, mental backwardness or bad environment. Unlike that passivity, which is a lack of a sense of work responsibility, laziness in school is greatly caused by the clash between the demands of the school and extra-curricular interests and it increases with age. By the 11th–12th year, one-third of the boys and a tenth of the girls are unable to reconcile their own interests with school work. The child is exclusively preoccupied with school only in the lowest primary grades.

For the pupil during puberty his interest and abilities, which now become specialized, and the type of school he attends, play a rôle that differs with each individual. The attitude of the adolescent to school is greatly influenced by practical or scientific interests, by the personality of the teacher which now becomes much more important than previously, and by his home environment. Several studies have contributed to an understanding of this problem. *Margarete Rada* [104] in a study of girls from the Viennese proletariat found that school plays a much greater rôle for them up to graduation, i.e. the fourteenth year, than for children from the middle classes because, for the proletariat children, school is practically the only place where they can find some intellectual stimulus, and a chance to discuss something besides daily cares about food and money. These girls therefore attend school very willingly. Twenty per cent of them are completely taken up with school and 70 per cent are quite enthusiastic about it. School remains the centre of their intellectual lives as long as they are not diverted from it by precocious sexual interests or the necessity to contribute to the support of their families. These girls whose interests are in the very nature of things non-intellectual, who give gymnastics and drawing as their favourite subjects, are well aware on the other hand of the importance of knowledge and evaluate the scientific subjects very highly.

Adolf Busemann [105] studied the rôle played by school during puberty for the higher grades. He attempted to establish which intellectual interest the school had aroused and how the students evaluated it. With the aid of a questionnaire, he tried to determine the rôle played by the school in creating, stimulating or decreasing their interests. Out of several hundred answers 66 per cent decided in favour of school as an influential factor. The results in detail are very revealing. Schools of the advanced types were considered as stimulating philological, historic and, surprisingly enough, also philosophic interest. But interest in natural science was not considered as being stimulated by school, although the majority of the students came from secondary schools in which special emphasis is placed on the natural sciences. School was further evaluated as not playing a very important rôle in relation to mechanical interests. The manner in which interests are aroused and strengthened varies with each subject. Whereas the teacher plays a decisive rôle in the study of the humanities since only he can transmit the content of a subject like language or history, or an enthusiasm for the antique cultures, in the study of the natural sciences, the student's own talents are of more importance. The positive contribution made by the higher institutions of learning, at any rate in Europe, consist, in the students' opinions, largely in arousing the student's appreciation of his cultural heritage rather than in developing intellectual powers for practical use.

Those students who found that the cultural influence of the school was very slight, held either the lack of any connection between the cultural subject and the actualities of existence or the lack of inspiring teachers responsible. This is certainly a decisive factor in shaping the cultural interest of the maturing student.

The specialization of interest and abilities goes hand in hand with the growing sense of independence and responsibility. *H. Busse* [106] has shown that by the eleventh year it becomes clear which of the students lean towards the natural sciences and which towards the arts. He bases his conclusions on questions asked spontaneously by the boys of his class.

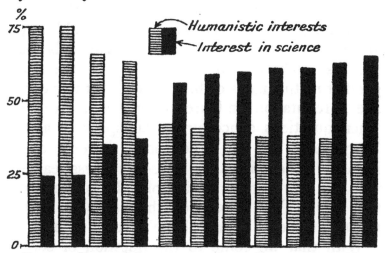

FIG. 17.—Types of Interest according to Busse, each double column representing the interests of one individual.

The development of special interest and abilities run parallel. We know from the preceding chapter that they do not appear before the 11th–12th year. This fact, which has been established by *Spearman,*[107] as we discussed in the foregoing chapter, and a number of other investigators, is advanced by the children themselves. A study of the first mention of special abilities made by students in a self-evaluation is under way in Vienna. It is surprising how few special abilities are mentioned in each class ; not more than 10 per cent of the pupils are described as highly talented, although many extra curricular activities like sports, music, dancing, etc., occur. Special talents are rarely mentioned before the eleventh year.

Observations made by *K. Reininger* [108] in an elementary school class of 11–12-year-old boys are of interest in this connection. He finds that the " specialists ", that is, those who are very good at mathematics or history, enjoy at this early age a reputation and are recognized as leaders when questions concerning their specialty arise. They never, on the other hand, become class leaders. Those boys are chosen as class leaders who are very popular and approach the ideal for that age. The leaders of the 11–12-year-olds must be good at sports above everything else.

With that we come to the question of social development in adolescence. Up to about the thirteenth year, both boys and girls are very sociable. Group life plays an important rôle. *Lucia Vecerka* [109] in a study of the friendships of girls found that the 11–12-year-olds were insatiable in their desire for friends. Friendships during that period are still somewhat superficial. *Lotte Danzinger* [110] studied the friendship of a group of 11–14-year-old working girls at an English camp. She describes them as follows :

> First of all a pair of friends are constantly together. One might imagine that they had quarrelled when by chance they were not together. With two exceptions this was never the case. Everything was done in the company of the friend ; eating, studying, playing, shopping, letter-writing and walking. All of those

activities could have been indulged in just as well, however, with many other girls; they in no way strengthened the personal bond between the two friends. The friendship was characterized by this tendency to do things together, as an end in itself. The wearing of similar clothes, the possession of similar things, bands and insignia.

They had little in common, and their being together was an end in itself. Phyllis, 11 ; 9, says of her friend, " She doesn't resemble me, but we always wear the same outfits, shoes and stockings." Dora, 11 ; 7, says, " We have often wished that we could wear the same clothes, but our mothers can't afford it." When sweets were distributed to the girls during an excursion, Marjorie, 11 ; 0, asked for a red candy. " Why do you want a red one ? "—" Oh, because Guenny also has a red one."

In the negative phase a radical change occurs. The youngster withdraws into himself, he is for a time definitely anti-social. He is unhappy without knowing why, and feels that no one understands his sufferings.

When this period of withdrawal has passed and social needs again concern the adolescent, they are of an entirely different nature than they were previously. The 15–18-year-old wants to find one single friend who understands him. It is interesting to observe how remarks made by these youngsters about their friends reveal the need for a deeper and more personal bond. *S. Roedleitner* [111] made a collection of the entries in the diaries of adolescents regarding their friends in order to ascertain statistically whether, as a rule, external events or emotional moments were mentioned in relation to a friend. She found the following distribution for the boys :

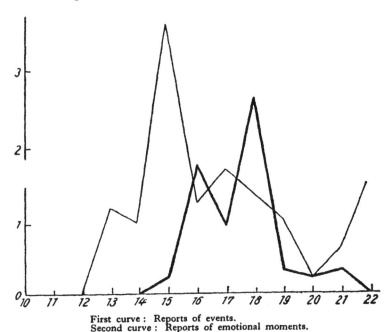

First curve : Reports of events.
Second curve : Reports of emotional moments.

FIG. 18.—Deepening of Friendships in the Case of Boys.

The need for mutual understanding and the sharing of ideas also furnishes the new basis for group organization during adolescence. *Lewis Martin* [112] was able to show that even in the political clubs friendships between the members were of more importance than the political ideology. A thorough discussion of adolescent group activities ranging from the " Kränzchen " and club to the degenerate " gang " form, that has been so authentically described by *F. Thrasher*,[113] would call for a chapter of its own. This would also be necessary for those clubs having a religious, moral or ideological basis. The reader can get an orientation in this field from other studies.[114]

In conclusion, a short description of the maturation of love and vocational attitudes will be presented.

By about the seventeenth year the individual matures in two spheres of paramount importance ; his love life and his work life. The setting up of criteria for maturity in these two essential trends of development is important because in dealing with neurotic, abnormal and delinquent adolescents we find as a rule that their development in one or both of these categories is defective.

Using the method of anamnesis, *Fritz Kolb and Maria Kostka* [114] investigated the development from the adolescent to the mature love phase and found that four steps are made before full maturity is reached. The first is the emotional devotion to another individual. In this early stage, from the fourteenth to the sixteenth year, this object of devotion may be an adult or another adolescent and may be a member of the same or of the opposite sex. This first devotion is not yet completely specific. The second step was called flirtation, and was defined as the first playful approach to the opposite sex. With the third and fourth step, the individual achieves physical sex maturity, and a degree of emotional maturity that is characterized by the ability and willingness to co-operate and form an entity with the partner. There are, then, two psychological steps, namely, the achievement of that degree of emotional readiness and of spiritual maturity that make the sharing of life problems with a partner possible, and two physical steps, the ability to make actual contact and to enter the sexual relationship. These four dispositions are the prerequisites for sexual maturity. In cases of sexual failure we are able to show where malformations have occurred. This is especially true in regard to neurotic or degenerate women. The difference between these two types is, namely, that the neurotic is inhibited in the consummation of the sexual act, whereas the degenerate shows defective emotional and mental reactions.

Maturity in the second major developmental step, i.e. in the field of work and vocation, is reached at about the seventeenth year. We distinguish here, following the detailed research made by *Paul Lazarsfeld*,[115] two essential attitudes as characteristic of maturity. The first attitude is characterized by the wish to achieve something. At about 17 the individual becomes dissatisfied, is no longer completely taken up with school work, and if already in a profession, suddenly not satisfied with the type of his activity so far. He wants to accomplish something that is as unique and significant as possible. In all the diaries that cover this phase we find this wish to do important work and to stand the test of responsibility.

The second aspect of work maturity expresses itself as the wish to reach a self-determined goal. It appears simultaneously with the wish to perform responsible tasks successfully, and is mentioned in almost every diary and conversation with individuals in this phase. At about 16 or 17 the individual begins for the first time to look at his life in retrospect, to give himself an account of his life to date, and to look forward into the future and decide what he ought to do. With the reaching of this level of self-determination we consider the transition from adolescence to maturity as accomplished.

CHAPTER X

THE INFLUENCE OF HEREDITY AND ENVIRONMENT ON THE DEVELOPMENT OF CHARACTER

WE have until now concerned ourselves with those facts of development that are largely independent of the individual situation. In the discussion of special abilities we paid no attention to the individually determined factors, but confined our investigation, with the exception of the study of individual cases and environmental influences in regard to pre-school children, to their chronological appearance. The older the child gets the more definitely do the effect of the influences exerted by the environment and the gradually crystallizing individuality of the child make their appearance. All of the investigations that we took up in the previous chapters indicate an intensification of special interests and abilities from about the eleventh to the twelfth year on. The same holds true for the specific personality of the individual. How and to what extent hereditary and environmental influences determine individuality is one of the most difficult problems in the entire field of psychology. Research in heredity on the one hand and in the environmental factor on the other, have begun to attack the problem from diametrically opposed angles. A third angle, typological research, which attempts to define individuality on the basis of constantly occurring characteristics, represents a point of view independent of the two just mentioned. A detailed discussion of these three points of view would take up an entire book. We will at this point present a few of those findings that are especially pertinent.

Most of the investigations that are concerned with inherited, typological and environmental influences in the school child are directed toward performance. *Wilhelm Peters* [116] was one of the first psychologists who made use of extensive statistical data in order to isolate inherited abilities as evidenced in family groups over several generations. His procedure consisted in comparing the school reports of 1,162 German country children with those of their 344 parents, 177 grandparents and 11 great-grandparents. He found the following correlation for general performance.

TABLE XVIII

CORRELATION OF PARENTS' AND CHILDREN'S SCHOOL
PERFORMANCES (AFTER PETERS)

Parents			Percentage of children whose performances were	
			Good	Poor
Good—good	.	.	77·0	25·0
Good—poor	.	.	59·7	40·3
Poor—poor	.	.	45·0	55·0

199

It is surprising that the more finely differentiated abilities show a relatively high correlation when one keeps in mind how great changes in pedagogic method have been within the last two or three generations. There is a high correlation between the reports of two generations as far as reading, writing and arithmetic are concerned. On the other hand, correlations for language, religion, manual training and singing show great inconsistencies.

Modern studies of the effect of the hereditary factor on intellectual performance have, with few exceptions, been made in England and in the United States. English investigators have been especially interested in the factor of heredity. A few of their most recent results follow: In one series of studies an attempt was made to trace the family tree of many children in a manner similar to that employed by *Peters* in Germany. *James Duff*,[117] for example, studied, among other things, the professions of the ancestors of children over a period of 130 years. It was found that more than twice as many fathers and grandfathers in this outstanding group were members of the higher professions than those in an average group that was used for comparison. In another series of studies a comparison was made between the home environment and the intellectual level of children who at an early age had been placed in orphan asylums or similar institutions. *E. M. Lawrence*,[118] in a thorough study, was able to establish a definite correlation between the performances of the children and their father's general cultural level. Those children whose fathers belonged to the two highest cultural groups, A and B, tested over a 100 ; those children from the progressively inferior environments, C, D and E, tested progressively from the 100 average to 92. In a third group of studies a comparison of intellectual performance was made for brothers and sisters, with special emphasis on twins. *Gesell's* work with twins belongs to this group. *Robert Davis* [119] found great similarities between the intellectual performances of brothers and sisters who from early childhood had been brought up in orphan asylums.

Very extensive are recent investigations of heredity in graphic, musical and mathematical talents.

Walter Krause, [120] under the direction of *W. Peters*, made an investigation in a small city in central Germany in which he studied 100 pairs of parents and their progeny in respect to drawing talent. He found that when both parents have more or less than average drawing talent, 75 to 90 per cent of the children's performances are of the same grade as the parents'. Where only one of the parents is talented the tendency is to take after the parent of the same sex. He also found that in drawing the males were consistently superior to the females, which also is clear from the fact that there is a higher talent correlation between talented sons and parents than between untalented daughters and parents. The fact that the variability of performance increases with increase in talent is of significance.

Theodor Ziehen and Valentin Haecker [121] carried out an investigation similar to *Krause's* of the inheritance of musical talent and later of its correlation with mathematical and drawing talent. They used a questionnaire that had been very carefully worked out and their results based on 1,000 questionnaires confirmed those of *Peters-Krause*. They also found that in discordant marriages when one parent was more talented than another, that their progeny show a greater leaning toward talent than away from it, the sons more than the daughters. Sixty per cent of the children have musical talent when one of the parents is talented. They also confirmed *Krause's* finding that there is a tendency to inherit a talent from the parent of the same sex with the exception that the sons of very highly gifted mothers show a tendency to take after them rather than the father.

In those marriages that show a positive concordance there is a positive inheritance that averages 75 to 80 per cent ; inheritance from the parent of the opposite sex about 5 per cent. The same as the findings of *Krause*. In those marriages that show a negative concordance only 55 per cent of the children showed a lack of talent :

highly gifted children were found in only 6 per cent of these marriages.

It must be kept in mind that in those cases where the child possesses talents that the parents lack, or vice versa, it would be necessary to include data for grandparents, since it is a *Mendelian* law that talent frequently skips a generation.

We have, then, arrived at quite exact conclusions regarding the inheritance of two of the outstanding forms of artistic talent, and have found that the percentage of cases for which inherited, and therefore innate dispositions play a deciding rôle in determining the direction that a talent takes is very high. It is clear, therefore, that there is such a thing as specifically inherited talent that manifests itself during the school age ; the percentage of pronounced cases in relation to the total population is not sufficient, however, to establish specific inherited abilities in large numbers, in the case of the average school child.

In studying special talents it is important to determine just what entities are innate and inherited. Research workers in this field have made some attempt to explain these connections. *Valentin Haecker* and *Theodor Ziehen*, whose very extensive study we have already mentioned, attempted also to determine the extent to which mathematical talent is inherited. They analysed and correlated the component elements present in mathematical talent. In other words, they did not begin with the assumption that mathematical talent is an indivisible unit, but split it up into its component elements, namely geometric-spatial and mathematical-logical thinking. They found that these two component parts showed a relatively high correlation. A divergence between digit memory and mental calculation occurred more frequently than between the two more specific components of mathematical talent mentioned above, and was also found in the inheritance of these abilities.

> G and L—that is, geometric-spatial and mathematical-logical components—show a higher correlation with each other than they do with C, that is, calculation. C can be plus when G and L are minus, but C is never entirely minus when G and L are plus. In positive and negative concordant marriages C shows a greater variation than G and L, whereas they have been demonstrated as inherited, that is, unitary in an investigation that, however, is statistically incomplete.

Mathematical talent is the only intellectual talent for which a talent unit and therefore hereditary transmissibility has with some degree of certainty been established. The talent entity is an important problem not only in regard to the inheritance of special abilities but also of defects. *Leta S. Hollingworth*,[122] in her book, *Special Talents and Defects*, which takes into account all of the available literature in the field, considers only the following activities as demonstrating special abilities and defects : reading and writing, mathematics, drawing and music. In reading and writing special defects which make their appearance in the earliest grades are of major importance. Mathematical ability is to date the only one of the special intellectual talents that has been clearly established as an entity.

Most of the investigations in this field during the last ten years or so have concentrated on the influence of environment on performance. American, English and German research workers have been especially active in this field. *A. Argelander* [123] presents a summary of the most important findings of those investigations. The following environmental factors were studied : profession of father, kind of home, size of family, family life. *Argelander* in a study of her own evaluated the environmental factors that had been established in previous studies, applying them to elementary school pupils from 7 to 15 years, and to the retarded pupils in special classes. She calculated an environment index from all the factors. In applying her index in a special study, she found an extraordinary difference of the environment index of retarded children compared with even a low class of elementary school children.

All investigators find again and again that the correlation between poor school work and home living conditions is especially high. In an interesting study of two groups of school-girls it was found by *Busemann and Bahr* [124] that an unemployment period for the father of not less than a year was reflected in the school work of the girls by a drop from the average school report of 2·82 to 3·13. This study is so much more pertinent than the simple correlation between environment and performance because the unfavourable effect of the change to a poorer environment can be followed in the same individuals.

A harmonious family life is another very important determinant for school performance. According to *Lämmermann's* [125] findings the correlation between school work and family income is 0·19, with the size of the family 0·32, with living conditions 0·53, with a harmonious family situation 0·63. This factor, which includes family quarrels, drunkenness, etc., exerts the most powerful influence of all on school performance. It has also been found that children from families lacking a parent show an inferiority in their school work.

The question of the rôle of the number of siblings and the order of birth has been largely investigated. *Busemann* [126] considered the group 2–3 siblings the most favourable situation. *Argelander*, on the other hand, showed that most investigators found that 1–2 siblings was the number most conducive to school success and that the incidence of poor performance was directly proportional to increase in sibling number. *Lentz* [127] showed that, on the average, families of two children showed a high incidence of unusual ability. There is a great difference of opinion about the favourable or unfavourable effect of the order of birth, that is, the position in the sibling series. Several American authors [128] claim that good school performance shows a high correlation with birth series position, i.e. the more recently born show better performance than the first-born. *Busemann*, on the other hand, finds that there is an 18 per cent incidence of school failure among first-born, 15 per cent for the middle born and 30 per cent for the last-born children. *Penrose* [129] finds the birth before the twenty-fifth year of the mother favourable. Also this question has been largely studied. It is clear, even from these few references, that school performance is influenced to a large extent by environmental factors.

In contradistinction to studies of heredity and environment which are directed toward the establishment of the causes of certain performances or defects, typological studies attempt to discover individual constants without inquiring into the causal factors. Following the lead of the typological studies of *Jung*,[130] *Kretschmer* [131] and *Jaensch*,[132] numerous attempts have been made to demonstrate typological differences as revealed in performance. Typological studies of children present as yet many difficulties in all probability because at this stage of the individual's development definite types seldom make their appearance.

The most exhaustive studies in this field have concerned themselves with perception, attention and richness or poverty of fantasy. The *Rhor-*

schach psychodiagnostic test was employed for investigating the latter. These experiments indicated that there are two types of mentality, one more abstract, logical, formal, the other more amorphous and interested in visual image and colour content. The latter type has strong social sympathies, is primitive, direct and very adaptable, whereas the former is unsocial, more complex, less adaptable.

Since those typological systems that have been established for adults have not as yet proved satisfactory in their application for children, the author attacked the problem of characterological study of children from a new angle. By means of this new method characterological constants were obtained by observing children over long periods of time. A limited number of children were studied. The reciprocal relationships between children and various individuals in a definite situation, namely in the family, and therefore the influence of the family on the child, as well as constant behaviour traits in the children, were studied in 20 families.

The following method is employed. A psychologist visits a family (twice a week) that is willing to have the children observed in the course of their daily routine. The visitor establishes a good contact with the family and makes herself generally useful by taking the children for walks, and helping them with their school work and around the house, etc. Outside of that she changes the natural family situation in no way. She is trained to record after her visit accurately the events that occur in the family during a one- to two-hour visit, so that a rough statistical evaluation of the material can be made. All of the behaviour units are counted and grouped according to various categories. It is possible as a result to present the relationship of the children to each other, of the children and parents to each other, and to set up a characterological profile of the child and family.

Up to the present time a series of typical basic situations constitute our main findings. The children live in a different basic situation depending on whether they are exposed to a loving, conscientious upbringing, intellectual or religious influences, or are exposed to discussions concerning household and business cares and family income. It also happens that in the same family the individual children have different basic situations as the two profiles that follow demonstrate. (See pages 210 and 211.)

The profiles are interpreted as follows : The behaviour responses and remarks of the parents of E. and K. are counted and arranged in six groups : Affection, care, upbringing, conversation, contact, play, household activities, etc. The profile shows how these varying types of behaviour are distributed.

It is clear from the situation profiles of K. and E. that they live in entirely different basic situations. Life in the family for Erna, who is 10 years old, consists mainly in meeting the demands of her environment. She has to help her mother

with the housework more than any of the other
children whom we observed. She gets no affection in return, the mother never plays with her,
she is not as well cared for physically as the

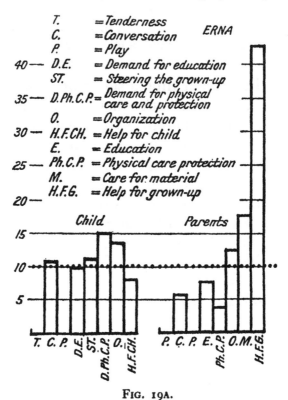

FIG. 19A.

FIGS. 19A and 19B.—Relationship

average of the children (which is seen from the
pointed horizontal line marking the average), and
her social needs and education are neglected.

Her sister, Käthe, who is 6 years old, is provided with an entirely different environment.

She is rarely asked to help her mother, although there is no servant. All these responsibilities are heaped on Erna's shoulders. In Käthe's case also the mother devotes very little time to play and

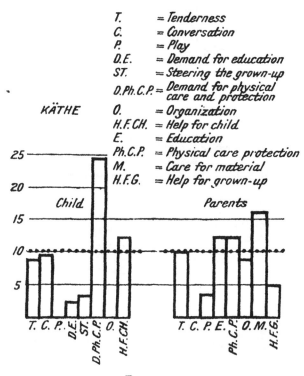

T.   = Tenderness
C.   = Conversation
P.   = Play
D.E.   = Demand for education
ST.   = Steering the grown-up
D.Ph.C.P. = Demand for physical care and protection
O.   = Organization
H.F.CH.   = Help for child
E.   = Education
Ph.C.P.   = Physical care protection
M.   = Care for material
H.F.G.   = Help for grown-up

FIG. 19B.
between Parents and their Two Girls.

social contact with the child. She is interested only in practical affairs, and as a result, Käthe, like her sister, hardly lives the life of a child, but is constantly involved in household affairs. But Käthe at any rate receives some tenderness from

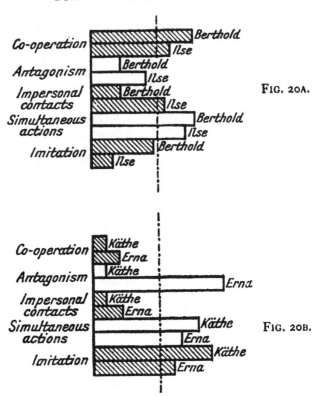

FIG. 20A.

FIG. 20B.

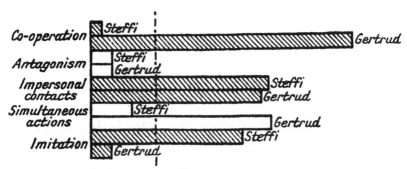

FIG. 20C.

FIGS. 20A, 20B and 20C.—Profiles of the Relationship between Three
Pairs of Siblings.

her parents and even a little more than the average physical care and educational opportunity, while Erna is left completely to herself in this respect. We find, then, that the basic situation in which the children grow up and which is designated as the characterological family profile is of decisive importance for character development. The behaviour profile of the children in their relationship to parents and siblings is determined by the basic situation. Let us now compare the following profiles for the relationship between the sisters Erna-Käthe and Gertrud-Steffi and a third pair of siblings, Ilse and Berthold.

These profiles were set up according to the degree of co-operation, antagonism, imitation, simultaneous activities and impersonal contacts which could be observed in the behaviour and the speech response between the siblings.

It is clear that the relationship between Käthe and Erna is coloured largely by Erna's antagonism to Käthe, while the character of the relationship between Gertrud and Steffi is the result of Gertrud's co-operative attitude. Steffi is also four years younger than her sister and is somewhat spoiled by her parents in comparison with the other sister. But since the basic family situation is the product of an affectionate parental attitude toward the children, it is transferred to the sister relationship. A third relationship between Ilse and Berthold gives us the example of a harmonious distribution of all possible contacts.

In continuing this investigation it will be necessary to establish the conditions that determine the various behaviour constants. We conclude our survey with the new possibilities that this research uncovers.[132a]

METHODS AND TECHNIQUES OF INVESTIGATION IN CHILD PSYCHOLOGY

THE carrying out of psychological experiments with children is beset with many difficulties. It is therefore important to decide at the outset which methods and techniques can furnish reliable data regarding the psychic life of the child. Modern child psychology makes use primarily of the methods of experimental conversation and observation. The latter, which has been precisely and systematically applied, has grown out of the method of incidental observation. *Wilhelm Preyer* [133] was the first to record observations of this nature in a diary that he kept of his own child. His work became a standard in the field and was followed by many imitators. Frequently mothers keep a day-book during the first year or two of a child's life and record behaviour that strikes them as especially interesting. What distinguishes these observations from the systematic recording of the modern psychologist ? The difference is best illustrated by the following examples. The first is taken from the diary that *Ernst* and *Gertrud Scupin*,[134] following *Preyer* as a model, and under the direction of *William Stern*, kept very carefully over a period of years of their son, Bubi.

Bubi, 4 weeks.
While asleep the child's clenched fists, with thumb between second and third finger, usually rest on its face.

APPENDIX

It enjoys pulling a serviette up over its face and snoring contentedly from underneath it. Tickling of the nose or eyebrows during sleep precipitated not the slightest defensive arm movement, in all probability because the sensitivity of the skin covering the face had been greatly reduced by the constant stimulation of the serviette. The child is easily frightened during sleep and often sighs uneasily. To-day we observed that it shuddered violently when the clock suddenly struck.

Let us now compare the above record with a systematic sleep observation such as we are accustomed to make nowadays : [135]

Time. 11 *months, 2 days.*

13.18 Eyes close, child sleeps.

13.20 A neighbouring child coughs, child opens eyes wide, shuts them at once and sleeps.

13.21 Opens eyes, babbles restlessly, twists head, one arm is drawn up against the chest, then outstretched ; lifts up cover repeatedly with legs. Moves head restlessly back and forth. Presses lips closely together, then separates them.

13.25 The eyes close. Head is turned to right (previously on left). The hands, slightly clenched, lie on each side of the head, the mouth is slightly open.

13.27 Eyelids slightly raised, then lowered.

13.29 Eyelids again slightly raised, turns head in sleep so that it lies straight back.

13.32 Opens eyes, yawns, turns head, stretches out hands, yawns, falls asleep.

13.36 Twists head, eyes are again open, hands move, child sleeps.

It will be obvious to the reader how the notation of the series of successive movements, accurately timed, has supplanted the rather vague, narrative formulation. *E.* and *G. Scupin* summarize occasionally observed details. For example : " the hands *usually* lie . . . the child *enjoys* doing this or that—the child *often* makes these sounds—

the child did this or that *to-day*." Our procedure, on the other hand, is to stand at the child's bedside for a given period of time, and make an accurate protocol of the child's total behaviour.

The question arises : how many of the countless movements of the child we can record, and to what extent we can describe them in detail ? The American behaviourists, and especially *John B. Watson*,[136] have theoretically been of the opinion that one must record each reflex, that is, each physiological unit of movement. This is a practical impossibility.

One can, it is true, describe the fright reaction of a new-born child to a very loud noise as *Watson* [136] does, for example : " . . . a jump, a start, a respiratory pause followed by more rapid breathing with marked vaso-motor changes, sudden closure of the eye, clutching of hands, puckering of lips " (page 152).

" A jump, a start," is not strictly speaking exact. Is it the head or the trunk that is pulled up, how high, how fast, etc. ? As one proceeds from the simple to the more complicated reactions it becomes increasingly diffi-cult to describe them accurately. Surprisingly enough, the descriptions of *Watson*, the most radical of the behaviourists, are from our point of view totally inac-curate. When he speaks of *smiling*, for example, he says :

Smiling : Smiling is due in all probability at first to the presence of kinaesthetic and actual stimuli. It appears as early as the fourth day. It can most often be seen after a full feeding. Light touches on parts of the body, blowing upon the body, touching the sex organs and sensitive zones of the skin are the unconditioned stimuli that will produce smiling. Tickling under the chin and a gentle jogging and rocking of the infant will often bring out smiling.

Smiling is the response in which conditioning factors begin to appear as early as the thirtieth day. Dr. Mary

APPENDIX

Cover Jones has made an extensive study of smiling. In a large group of children she found that conditioned smiling —that is, smiling when the experimenter smiles or says babyish words to the infant (both auditory and visual factors)—begins to appear at around the thirtieth day. In her total study of 183 cases, the latest age at which the conditioned smile first appeared was 80 days (page 122).

This description is highly inaccurate. It is first of all necessary that those facial movements that we are to consider " smiling " be accurately established. The first primitive attempts to draw up the corners of the mouth, described by *Preyer* as the sequel to a satisfying meal observed in the newly-born infant, differs radically from the drawing up of the mouth accompanied by a sparkling of the eyes that we can observe as a response to the human voice or glance from the fourth week of life.[137] In descriptions of this nature accuracy is of the greatest importance, because the expressions of satisfaction are fundamentally different from those of smiling. The first follows a state of physical satisfaction, the second is primarily the result of the psychological effect of another person. Smiling in response to the touching of the body, tickling, or other kinaesthetic or tactile stimuli has not been observed in the new-born child prior to smiling in response to another human being. Therefore, *Watson* comes to a false conclusion.

We expect and achieve, in our observations of behaviour, a much greater accuracy and refinement of registration than *Watson*. And it is possible that just because our observations are actually much more exact than those of the theoretical behaviourists, we realize that recording in reflexological terms is an impossible goal for psychology. Reflexes are physiological units. The psychological unit, on the other hand, is performance or achievement, that is, an event that has a definite significance and result. An example follows :

> Under the direction of *Lois Hayden Meek, Dorothy Swaine Thomas* [138] has worked out techniques of protocolling, taking the extreme behaviouristic point of view. It is maintained that in her work, *Resistant Behaviour of Preschool Children, R. K. Caille* [139] describes unruly children following these techniques. One of her description units is : " Larry has a tin pan. Spencer pulls at it. Larry pulls back, keeps it (this is an instance of what we term ' successful resistance '), and says, ' I need it.' "

The recorded unit here is " pulls back, keeps it ". It is in no sense a reflex, but rather a series of movements, such as, child moves arm over its own body, grabs an object with its hand, strong contractions, etc. In addition, the description " pulling towards self, and holding fast " involves much more than just a movement towards the grasping of an object. The fact that an object is held fast or taken away from some one includes in addition a specific significance and result, and it is exactly this significance and result that distinguishes this behaviour from a series of physiological reflexes. No matter how carefully all the reflexes, the rapidity and angle of movements, etc., are described, no one could possibly know that in this case, not only was an object grasped, but kept, and that it was not only drawn close, but actively defended. There are, notwithstanding, certain complexes of behaviour that we can analyse down into movements which constitute a performance unit. An example follows :

> *Olga Rubinow and Liselotte Frankl* [140] have made very exact studies of the infant in the earliest feeding situation and of the reactions following the perception of the bottle. A white wooden cone with the apex directed toward the

child (4 months) precipitated a reaction that is described as follows :
Looks at the point for some time.
Body is tense.
Breathes rapidly.
Opens mouth.
Kicks vigorously.
We can deduce from this protocol that the child mistakes the wooden cone that is brought close to its mouth for its bottle, since it reacts exactly with the same movements when being offered the bottle. The fact that the infant of this age recognizes the bottle as yet only from the point that is moved towards it is responsible for this inadequate reaction. We have succeeded in reducing the act " recognizing of bottle " to the component movements that are always present when this child reacts to its bottle. We can therefore establish the behaviour unit " recognizing of bottle " from the complex of its constituent individual movements.

For the psychologist the point of departure must be the behaviour unit. He wishes to determine whether or not the child recognizes the bottle. It is only in connection with the recognition of the bottle that he is interested in the child's breathing and impulsive movements. Not these acts in themselves, but their why and wherefore are his problem. Exact observations of specific behaviour units is the method *par excellence* in child psychology.

Generally, the observation is an experimental one. Under experiment we define a planned modification of the normal life situation of the child that is undertaken for research purposes. The simplest form of experiment, for instance, would be the presentation of a toy to a child and the observation of its subsequent reaction. The experiments that are employed in child psychology are such simple variations of the natural life situation of the child. Apparatus and laboratory situations are avoided as far as possible because we know that circumstances as artificial as these distort the child's natural reactions. Scientists like *Arnold Gesell*,[141] who work with children under laboratory conditions, take great pains to accustom the child to these situations over a period of days or weeks in order that the child shall behave naturally. It is as yet a matter of debate whether or not this can actually be achieved.

In addition to the experiment which can be used with care at all age-levels, there is also the method of the oral or written questionnaire, which is in the main applicable to older children. *Jean Piaget* [142] has of late had considerable success with this method in the form of exploratory conversations. Experience would indicate that valuable insights can be gained from conversations with children as early as the fifth year. The written questionnaire method is as a matter of course usable only from school age on, and it is being replaced more and more by the oral questionnaire. Exploratory conversations with parents and teachers concerning the children whom they have observed is a new method used by *Anderson* and *Goodenough* [143]—recently by *Mary Shirley* [144] and by *Liselotte Frankl* [145] with conspicuous success.

REFERENCES

[1] Page 1. W. BECHTEREW, *New Studies in the Reflexology and Physiology of the Nervous System.* (Russian) 1925.

[2] Page 1. A. GESELL, *The Mental Growth of the Pre-School Child.* N.Y., 1925.

[3] Page 4. CH. BÜHLER, *The First Year of Life.* N.Y., 1930.

[4] Page 3. "Day Circles" taken from the book CH. BÜHLER, *Kindheit und Jugend.* Leipzig (Hirzel), 3rd edition, 1931. See also *The First Year of Life.*

[5] Page 6. See E. B. WARING and M. WILKER, *The Behaviour of Young Children.* N.Y., 1929.

[5a] Page 6. Y. KAMIMURA, "Ueber den Schlaf im Kindesalter, Jido-Kenkyn," *Japan, Ztschr. für Kinderkunde*, **136**. Tokio, 1932.

[5b] Page 6. E. ANDERSON, J. FOSTER and F. GOODENOUGH, The Sleep of Young Children, *J. Gen. Ps.*, **35**, 1928.

[6] Page 10. CH. BÜHLER and H. HETZER, *Testing Children's Development.* London (Allen & Unwin), 1935.

[6a] Page 16. See M. WOLF, "Developmental Tests with Well-to-do Children," *A. Ges. Ps.* In Print.

[7] Page. 16. O. RUBINOW and L. FRANKL are working out in Vienna these test devices.

[8] Page 20. See reference 6a.

[8a] Page 20. L. TERMAN, *Genetic Studies of Genius.* 3 Vols. Stanford Univ. Press.

[8b] Page 20. M. SHIRLEY, *The First Two Years.* 3 vols. Univ. of Minnesota Press, 1933.

[9] Page 35. L. DANZINGER and L. FRANKL, "Zum Problem der Funktionsreifung; Entwicklungsprüfungen an albanischen Kindern," *Z. Kif.*, **43**, 1934.

[10] Page 36. M. B. McGRAW applied our tests to Negro infants. See *A Comparative Study of a Group of Southern White and Negro Infants*, Gen. Ps. Mon., **10**. Worcester, 1931.

REFERENCES

[11] Page 57. CH. BÜHLER, " Soziale Verhaltungsweisen im ersten Lebensjahr," *Qu. Stud. Jugdk.*, **5**, Jena, 1927. A continuation of these studies is with more details, discussion of literature and methods in preparation, by L. BERG and M. MAUDRY.

[11a] Page 64. J. K. FRIEDJUNG, *Die kindliche Sexualität.* Berlin, 1923.

[11b] Page 64. C. BOENHEIM, *Kinderpsychotherapie in der Praxis.* Berlin, 1932.

[11c] Page 64. See the detailed discussion of this problem in CH. BÜHLER, " Zum Problem der sexuellen Entwicklung," *Z. Kihlkde*, **51**, 1931.

[12] Page 66. R. KLEIN, " Die Autorität als eine Form der sozialen Beeinflussung," *Z. Kif.*, **39**, 1932.

[13] Page 69. E. BENJAMIN, *Grundlagen und Entwicklungsgeschichte der kindlichen Neurose.* Leipzig, 1930.

[13a] Page 69. F. GOODENOUGH, *Anger in Young Children.* Minneapolis, 1931.

[13b] Page 74. E. KÖHLER, *Die Persönlichkeit des Dreijährgen.* Leipzig, 1926.

[14] Page 76. J. PIAGET, *Le langage et la pensée.* Neuchâtel, Paris, 1923.

[15] Page 77. H. M. HALVERSON, *An Experimental Study of Prehension in Infants*, Gen. Ps. Mon., **10**. Worcester, 1931.

[16] Page 78. E. DANIELS and M. MAUDRY, " Abwehrreaktionen auf Hindernisse bei Säuglingen", *Z. Ps.* In Print.

[17] Page 81. See H. HETZER, " Kind und Schaffen," *Qu. Stud. Jgdk.*, **7**, 1931.

[18] Page 84. See reference 9.

[19] Page 88. A. GESELL and H. THOMPSON, *Learning and Growth in Identical Twins*, Gen. Ps. Mon., **6**. Worcester, 1929.

[20] Page 89. M. McGRAW. See report in *Science News Letter*, **24**, 1933.

[21] Page 89. F. R. HILGARD, " Learning and Maturation in Preschool Children," *J. Gen. Ps.*, **41**, 1933.

[22] Page 90. A. JERSILD, *Training and Growth in the Development of Children*, Child Dev. Mon., **10**, New York, 1932.

[23] Page 91. O. MARUM and I. JASKULSKI, " Untersuchun-

REFERENCES

gen über die Stellung des Kindes zu sich selbst.," *Z. Kif.*, **41**, 1933.

[24] Page 93. L. FARWELL, *Reactions of Kindergarten-, First- and Second-Grade Children to Constructive Play Materials*, Gen. Ps. Mon., **8**, 1930.

[25] Page 98. F. BEYRL, "Ausdauer und Konzentration im Vorschulalter ", *Z. Ps.*, **107**, 1928.

[26] Page 98. H. SHACTER, "A Method for Measuring Sustained Attention of Preschool Children ", *J. Gen. Ps.*, **42**, 1933.

[27] Page 100. H. VOLKELT, "Das bildnerisch gestaltende Kind ". (I) M. MÜSSLER, "Das Bauen des Kindes mit zweifarbigem Material", *Neue Ps. Stud.*, **8**. München, 1933.

[28] Page 100. H. HETZER. In preparation.

[29] Page 106. See reference 9.

[30] Page 107. K. BÜHLER, *Sprachtheorie*. Jena, 1934.

[31] Page 108. K. BÜHLER, *Die geistige Entwicklung des Kindes*. 6. Aufl., Jena, 1930.

[32] Page 109. M. BERGEMANN-KÖNITZER, "Das plastische Gestalten des Kleinkindes ", *Z. Ang. Ps.*, **31**, 1928.

[33] Page 110. E. HANFMANN, "Ueber das Bauen der Kinder ", *Z. Kif.*, **36**, 1930.

[34] Page 111. O. KRAUTTER, "Die Entwicklung des plastischen Gestaltens beim vorschulpflichtigen Kind," Beih. 50, *Z. Ang. Ps.* 1930.

[35] Page 119. L. DANZINGER, "Schulreifetests ", *Wiener päd. Ps.*, **9**, 1933.

[36] Page 121. A. ADLER, *Ueber den nervösen Charakter*, 3. Aufl., München, 1922. *Studien über Minderwertigkeit von Organen*. 2. Aufl., München, 1927.

[37] Page 121. P. LAZARSFELD, *Die körperliche und geistige Entwicklung*. Quelle 79. Wien, 1929.

[38] Page 122. A. NETSCHAJEFF, "Psychologische Untersuchungen bei Kindern im Alter von 4-8 Jahren ", *Z.a.P.* **29**, 1928.

[39] Page 122. E. LIEFMANN, "Volksschülerinnen, ihre geistigen und körperlichen Leistungen und deren Beziehung zur Konstitution ", *Z.a.P.*, **43**, 1932. "Ueber geistige und körperliche Leistungen von Repetenten," *Z. päd. Ps.*, **34**, 1933.

REFERENCES

[40] Page 123. L. S. HOLLINGWORTH, *Gifted Children*. N.Y., 1926.

[41] Page 123. R. L. SANDWICH, " Correlation of Physical Health and Mental Efficiency ", *J. Educ. Ps.*, 1920.

[41a] Page 125. O. DECROLY, *Etudes de psychogénèse*. Bruxelles, 1932.

[42] Page 127. P. GREENBERG, " Competition in Children ", *Amer. J. of Ps.*, 44, 1932.

[42a] Page 128. A. L. EMMONS, " A Study of the Relation between Self-assurance and Skill in Young Children ", *Child Dev.*, 4, 1933.

[43] Page 128. H. HETZER and H. WINKOWSKI. Not yet published.

[43a] Page 129. M. E. SMITH, " The Pre-school Child's Use of Criticism ", *Child Dev.*, 3, 1932.

[43b] Page 129. H. HETZER and E. PODELIL. Not yet published.

[44] Page 131. J. C. FOSTER, " Verbal Memory in the Preschool Children ", *J. Gen. Ps.*, 35, 1928. See for more literature in this field, BUFORD JOHNSON, *Child Psychology*. Baltimore and London, 1933.

[45] Page 132. C. A. PROBST, " A General Information Test for Kindergarten Children ", *J. Child Devel.*, 1931.

[46] Page 132. H. P. DAVIDSON, *An Experimental Study of Bright, Average and Dull Children*. Gen. Ps. Mon., 9, 1932.

[47] Page 133. J. P. DRISCOLL, *The Development of the Preschool Child*. Child. Dev. Mon., 13, 1933.

[48] Page 133. See reference 38.

[49] Page 133. L. C. STRAYER, *Language and Growth*, Gen. Ps. Mon., 8, 1933.

[50] Page 134. E. KAWOHL, " Die kindliche Frage ", *Vitljschr. f. wissl. Päd.*, 4. Münster, 1929.

[51] Page 134. J. PIAGET, *Le langage et la pensée*, Paris, 1923.

[51a] Page 135. M. K. PYLER, " Verbalization as a Factor in Memory ", *J. Child Dev.*, 3, 1932.

[52] Page 135. USNADZE, " Begriffsbildung im vorschulpflichtigen Alter," *Z.a.P.*, 34, 1929.

[53] Page 136. J. PIAGET, *La représentation du monde chez l'enfant*. Paris, 1926.

REFERENCES

[53a] Page 138. See 31.

[53b] Page 138. W. MENAKER, " Furcht und Neugier in den ersten zwei Lebensjahren ", *Z. Ps.* In Print.

[53c] Page 138. S. ISAACS, *Intellectual Growth in Young Children.* London, 1930.

[53d] Page 139. S. WISLITZKY, " Gruppenbildung im Kindergarten ", *Z. Ps.*, **107**, 1928.

[54] Page 140. H. HETZER, " Das volkstümliche Kinderspiel ", *Wiener päd. Ps.*, **6**, 1927.

[55] Page 140. KARL REININGER, " Das soziale Verhalten der Schulneulinge ", *Wiener päd. Ps.*, **7**, 1929.

[56] Page 143. See reference 13.

[57] Page 144. Vienna study in preparation for publication.

[58] Page 144. A. BUSEMANN, *Die Jugend im eigenen Urteil.* Langensalza, 1926.

[59] Page 144. H. HETZER, " Das grossprecherische Kind ", *Päd. Warte*, **37**, 1930.

[60] Page 144. K. REININGER, " Soziale Verhaltungsweisen in der Vorpubertät, *Wiener päd. Ps.*, **2**, 1925.

[61] Page 145. E. MENAKER, F. SACK, L. DANZINGER. In preparation for publication.

[62] Page 152. E. BRUNSWIK, L. GOLDSCHEIDER, E. PILEK, *Untersuchungen zur Entwicklung des Gedächtnisses*, Beih. 64, *Z.a.P.*, 1932.

[63] Page 153. E. KÖHLER and I. HAMBERG, *Zur Psych. u. Pädag. der geistigen Aktivität.* Berlin, 1931.

[64] Page 153. A. HERRMANN, " Die Fähigkeit zu selbständigem Lernen," *Z. Ps.*, **109**, 1928.

[65] Page 154. E. KÖHLER, *Entwicklungsgemässer Schaffensunterricht.* Wien, 1932.

[66] Page 155. C. HELWING. See reference 2.

[67] Page 155. H. HETZER, *Schüler und Schulzeugnis.* Leipzig, 1933.

[68] Page 156. F. HOPPE und K. LEWIN, " Erfolg und Misserfolg," *Ps. Forschung*, **14**, 1930.

[69] Page 157. M. KEILHACKER, *Der ideale Lehrer nach der Aeusserung der Schüler.* Freiburg, 1932.

[70] Page 158. See reference 137.

[71] Page 160. W. PETERS, in his article " Begabungsprobleme " (*Z. päd. Ps.*, **26**, 1925) shows the consequences of the

REFERENCES

fact that the term " talent " is not a scientific one, but taken from practical life.

[72] Page 160. W. STERN, *Intelligenz der Kinder und Jugendlichen.* 4. Aufl. Leipzig, 1929.

[73] Page 160. W. PETERS, " Das Intelligenzproblem und die Intelligenzforschung ", *Z. Ps.*, **89**, 1922.

[74] Page 160. E. L. THORNDIKE, *Educational Psychology.* 3 vols. New York, 1903–13.

[75] Page 161. C. SPEARMAN, *The Abilities of Man, Their Nature and Measurement.* London, 1927.

[75a] Page 161. C. BURT, " The Mental Differences between Individuals," Report of the Brit. Assoc., 1923, " The Measurement of Mental Capacities," Henderson Trust Lecture, 1927. *The Distribution and Relations of Educational Abilities*, 1917.

[75b] Page 161. W. BROWN and G. H. THOMPSON, *The Essentials of Mental Measurement*, 1925. See the intelligent report of H. WYNN JONES, " Theories of intellectual factors ", *Brit. J. of Educ. Psych.*, **3**, 1933.

[75c] Page 163. J. B. RUSSELL, " The Relation of Intellectual, Temperamental and other Qualities to success in School ", *Brit. J. Ps.*, **24**, 1933–4.

[76] Page 163. K. MARBE and L. SELL, " Die Abhängigkeit der Schulleistung vom Lebensalter und Milieu ", *Z. Ps.*, **122**, 1931.

[77] Page 164. F. BRAUN, " Vom Einfluss des Schulalters auf die Schulleistungen ", *Arch. ges. Ps.*, **70**, 1929.

[78] Page 165. C. BURT, *Mental and Scholastic Tests.* London, 1921.

[79] Page 165. H. LÄMMERMANN, " Das Verhältnis von Allgemein- und Sonderbegabung, auf der Oberstufe der Volksschule ", *Z. päd. Ps.*, **34**, 1933.

[80] Page 166. STANTON and KOERTH, *Musical Capacity Measures of Children, Univ. of Iowa Studies*, **42**, 1933.

[81] Page 166. C. HAECKER and TH. ZIEHEN, " Die Erblichkeit der musikalischen Begabung ", *Z. Ps.*, **88–90**, 1922.

[82] Page 167. A. NESTLE, " Die musikalische Produktion im Kindesalter ", Beih. **52**, *Z.a.P.*, 1931.

[83] Page 167. O. REIMERS, " Untersuchungen über die Entwicklung des Tonalitätsgefühles im Laufe der Schulzeit ", *Z.a.P.*, **28**, 1927.

REFERENCES

[84] Page 167. G. Révész, "Prüfung der Musikalität," *Z. Ps.*, **85**, 1920.

[85] Page 168. F. Prager, "Experimentell-psychologische Untersuchungen über rhythmische Leistungsfähigkeit im Kindesalter," *Z.a.P.*, **26**, 1926.

[86] Page 168. H. Meier and G. Pfahler, "Untersuchung des technisch-praktischen und des technisch-theoretischen Verhaltens bei Schulkindern", *Z.a.P.*, **27**, 1926.

[87] Page 169. V. Neubauer, "Ueber die Entwicklung der technischen Begabung", *Z.a.P.*, **27**, 1926.

[88] Page 170. See the quotations from Karl Bühler, *Geistige Entwicklung des Kindes*, 6. Aufl., Jena, 1930.

[89] Page 171. See No. 13[b].

[90] Page 171. F. Baumgarten, *Wunderkinder*. Leipzig, 1933.

[91] Page 172. M. Whitley, "Children's Interests in Collecting ", *J. of Educ. Ps.*, **20**, 1929.

[92] Page 172. H. Lehmann and P. Witty, "The Present Status of the Tendency to Collect and Hoard ", *Ps. Rev.*, **34**, 1927. "Further Studies of Children's Interests in Collecting ", *J. of Educ. Ps.*, **21**, 1930. "The Collecting Interests of Town Children and Country Children ", *J. of Educ. Ps.*, **24**, 1933.

[92a] Page 172. W. F. Durost, "Children's Collecting Activity Related to Social Factors ", *Col. Univ. T. C. Contributions to Educ.*, **535**, 1932.

[93] Page 173. L. Danzinger. In preparation.

[94] Page 174. G. Scupin, *Lebensbild eines deutschen Schuljungen*. Leipzig, 1931.

[95] Page 182. H. Hetzer, "Soziale Verhaltungsweisen von Mädchen ", *Qu. Stud. Jdk.*, **4**, Jena, 1926.

[96] Page 182. See No. 11[a].

[97] Page 182. C. Boenheim, "Zur Frage der Onanie im Kindesalter ", *Dtsche. med. Wochschr.*, **47**, 1928.

[98] Page 182. S. Freud, *Drei Abhandlungen zur Sexualtheorie*, 6. Aufl. Berlin, 1926.

[99] Page 182. M. Hirschfeld, *Sexualpathologie*. 1917.

[100] Page 182. Meirowski-Neisser, *Das Geschlechtsleben der Jugend*. Schule und Elternhaus, 1912.

[100a] Page 183. O. Schwarz, *Sexualität und Persönlichkeit*. Leipzig und Wien, 1934.

REFERENCES

[101] Page 187. E. R. JAENSCH, *Ueber den Aufbau der Wahrnehmungswelt und die Eidetik.* 2. Aufl. Leipzig, 1927.

[102] Page 187. O. KROH, *Subjektive Anschauungsbilder bei Jugendlichen.* Göttingen, 1922.

[103] Page 187. P. P. BLONSKY, "Die faulen Schüler," *Z. Kif.*, 36, 1930.

[104] Page 188. M. RADA, "Das reifende Proletariermädchen". *Wiener Arb. z. päd. Ps.*, 83, 1932.

[105] Page 189. A. BUSEMANN, "Interesse an geistigen Gegenständen, etc.", *A.f.ges.Ps.*, 83, 1932.

[106] Page 190. H. H. BUSSE, *Kinder fragen den Lehrer.* Leipzig, 1931.

[107] Page 191. C. SPEARMAN, see reference 75.

[108] Page 192. K. REININGER, "Das soziale Verhalten in der Vorpubertät", *Wi. pä. Ps.*, 2, 1925.

[109] Page 192. L. VECERKA, Soziales Verhalten von Mädchen., *Qu. Stud. Jgdk.*, 4, Jena, 1926.

[110] Page 192. L. DANZINGER. See CH. BÜHLER, *Kindheit und Jugend*, pages 326 f.

[111] Page 193. S. ROEDLEITNER. See CH. BÜHLER, *Kindheit und Jugend*, pages 369 f.

[112] Page 194. L. MARTIN. See CH. BÜHLER, *Kindheit und Jugend*, pages 365 f.

[113] Page 195. F. THRASHER, *The Gang.* Chicago, 1927.

[114] Page 195. See CH. BÜHLER, *Kindheit und Jugend.* CH. BÜHLER, *Das Seelenleben des Jugendlichen.* 5. Aufl. Jena, 1930. *Diaries of Adolescents* (in preparation).

[115] Page 196. P. LAZARSFELD, "Jugend und Beruf", *Qu. Stud. Jgdk.*, 8, Jena, 1931.

[116] Page 199. W. PETERS, "Ueber Vererbung psychischer Fähigkeiten", *Fortschritte der Psychologie*, 3, 1915.

[117] Page 200. J. F. DUFF, "Children of High Intelligence, a Following-up Inquiry", *Brit. J. Ps.*, 19, 1928–9.

[118] Page 200. E. M. LAWRENCE, "An Investigation into the Relation between Intelligence and Inheritance", *Brit. J. Ps.*, Suppl. 11, 1931.

[119] Page 201. R. A. JR. DAVIS, "The Influence of Heredity on Mentality of Orphan Children", *Brit. J. Ps.*, 19, 1928–9.

REFERENCES

[120] Page 201. W. KRAUSE, " Experimentelle Untersuchungen über die Vererbung der zeichnerischen Begabung ", *Z. Ps.*, **126**, 1932.

[121] Page 202. TH. ZIEHEN and V. HAECKER, " Erblichkeit der musikalischen Begabung ", *Z. Ps.*, **88–90**, 1922. " Beitrag zur Lehre von der Vererbung und Analyse der zeichnerischen und mathematischen Begabung, insbesondere mit Bezug auf die Korrelation zur musikalischen Begabung ", *Z. Ps.*, **120–1**, 1931.

[122] Page 204. L. S. HOLLINGWORTH, *Special Talents and Defects*. New York, 1923.

[123] Page 205. A. ARGELANDER, " Die Bedeutung des Milieus für die intellektuelle Entwicklung ", *Hdb. der päd. Milieukunde*, herg. v. Busemann, Halle, 1932. " Der Einfluss der Umwelt auf die geistige Entwicklung ", *Jenaer Beitrge f. J. u. Erz. Ps.*, **7**, Langensalza, 1928.

[124] Page 205. BUSEMANN-BAHR, " Arbeitslosigkeit und Schulleistungen ", *Z. päd. Ps.*, **32**, 1931.

[125] Page 206. H. LÄMMERMANN, " Das Verhältnis von Allgemein-und Sonderbegabung auf der Oberstufe der Volksschule ", *Z. päd. Ps.*, **34**, 1933.

[126] Page 206. A BUSEMANN, " Geschwisterschaft und Schulzensuren ", *Z. Kif.*, **34**, 1928.

[127] Page 206. LENTZ, JR., " Relation of I.Q. to Size of Family ", *J. of Educ. Ps.*, **18**, 1927.

[128] Page 207. See L. L. THURSTONE and R. L. JENKINS, " Birth Order and Intelligence ", *J. of Educ. Ps.*, **20**, 1929.
M. L. STECKEL, " Intelligence and Birth Order in Families ", *J. of Soc. Ps.*, **1**, 1930.
G. ARTHUR, " The Relation of I.Q. to Position in Family ", *J. of Educ. Ps.*, **17**, 1926.

[129] Page 207. L. S. PENROSE, " A Study in the Inheritance of Intelligence ", *Brit. J. Ps.*, **24**, 1933.

[130] Page 207. C. G. JUNG, *Psychologische Typen*, Zürich, 1921.

[131] Page 207. E. KRETSCHMER, *Körperbau und Charakter*. 4. Aufl. Berlin, 1925.

REFERENCES

[132] Page 207.   E. R. Jaensch, "Verhältnis der Integrations-typologie zur Typenlehre Kretschmers ", *Z. Ps.*, **125**, 1932.
See also G. Pfahler, " System der Typen-lehre ", Ergbd. 15, *Z. Ps.*, 1929.

[132a] Ch. Bühler is preparing, with L. Danzinger, G. Falk, S. Gedeon, E. N. Ryan, several publications on this subject. The first book, *Child and Family*, will be edited with Harper & Br., New York, in the coming fall.

[133] Page 215.   W. Preyer, *Die Seele des Kindes.*   7. Aufl. Leipzig, 1908.

[134] Page 215.   E. u. G. Scupin, *Bubis erste Kindheit.* Leipzig, 1907.

[135] Page 216.   See Ch. Bühler und H. Hetzer, " Inventar der Verhaltungsweisen des ersten Lebensjahres ", *Qu. Stud. Jgdk.*, **5**, Jena, 1927.

[136] Page 217.   J. B. Watson, *Behaviourism*, 2nd Edn., London, 1931.

[137] Page 218.   See Ch. Bühler und H. Hetzer, reference 135, and H. Hetzer and B. Tudor-Hart, " Die früheste Reaktion auf die menschliche Stimme ", *Qu. Stud. Jgdk.*, **5**, 1927.

[138] Page 219.   D. S. Thomas, *Some New Techniques for Studying Social Behaviour.*   Ch. Dev. Mon., **1**.   New York, 1923.

[139] Page 219.   R. K. Caille, *Resistant Behaviour of Pre-school Children.*   Ch. Dev. Mon., **13**.   New York, 1933.

[140] Page 219.   O. Rubinow and L. Frankl, " Die erste Dingauffassung beim Säugling ", *Z.P.*, **133**, 1934.

[141] Page 221.   Compare in the Genetic Ps. Mon., Clark University Press, Worcester, the later studies which have been made under Arnold Gesell in The Yale University Psycho-Clinic.

[142] Page 221.   See the above-mentioned references, Nos. 14, 51, 53.

[143] Page 221.   J. Anderson and F. Goodenough, *Experi-mental Child Study.*   New York, 1931.

[144] Page 221.   M. Shirley.   See No. 8b.

[145] Page 221.   L. Frankl, " Die Anwendung von Lohn und Strafe in Familien ", *Qu. Stud. Jgdk.*, **12**, 1935.

INDEX OF SUBJECTS

INDEX OF SUBJECTS

INDEX OF SUBJECTS

INDEX OF SUBJECTS